Nursing
Diagnosis

CARE
PLANS

D0365874

NURSING DIAGNOSIS
POCKET GUIDE

Nursing
Diagnosis

CARE
PLANS

VELMA C. FREY, RN
President, Progressive Registered Nursing
Newberg, Oregon

CHRISTINE HOCKETT, RN, BSN
Nursing Supervisor, Newberg Community Hospital
Newberg, Oregon

GERRI MOIST, RN
ICU Nurse, St. Vincent's Hospital
Portland, Oregon

WILLIAMS & WILKINS
Baltimore • London • Los Angeles • Sydney

Copyright © 1986
Williams & Wilkins
428 East Preston Street
Baltimore, MD 21202, U.S.A.

Printed in the United States of America

First Edition,

Library of Congress Cataloging in Publication Data

Main entry under title:

Frey, Velma C.
  Nursing diagnosis care plans.

  "A Nurseco book."
  Bibliography: p.
  Includes index.
  1. Diagnosis. 2. Nursing care plans. 3. Diagnosis related groups. I. Hockett, Christine. II. Moist, Gerri. III. Title. [DNLM: 1. Nursing Process. 2. Patient Care Planning. WY 100 F893n]
RT48.F74   1986   610.73   86-4091
ISBN 0-683-09556-0

86 87 88 89 90   10 9 8 7 6 5 4 3 2 1

To my husband, Tom, and sons, Tom and David,
thank you.

V.C.F.

To my own dear Gene and Betty May,
who challenge me, encourage me, and believe in
me.

C.H.

To my family with love. Thanks for the patience
and support!

G.M.

Foreword   The quantification of nursing, although often attempted, has never been achieved in any workable standard format. The current climate of our nation's health care delivery system has made it apparent that this goal must be attained.

With the inception of the federal government's prospective payment system, the hospital industry is finding itself under a microscope: each service is being dissected and analyzed for efficiency, cost effectiveness, and quality.

DRGs (Diagnosis Related Groups) are the basis on which the payment system will operate. By themselves, DRGs are a tool to measure medical care consumed by hospitalized patients. They are also, however, the system by which hospitals receive reimbursement. Therefore any effort to quantify nursing or any other hospital service must include an interface with DRGs.

For many years nursing care plans were the keystone of nursing care. Based on theoretical models, they incorporated the assessment, planning, implementation, and evaluation processes of nursing care and provided a communication link between nurses and others involved in patient care. They also served as a guide for formulating nursing notes and goal setting.

More recently, nursing diagnoses have been designed to standardize the nomenclature and clearly identify the unique contribution of nursing to patient care. When properly utilized, they clarify roles by defining those activities that are the responsibility of the nurse.

Each tool—DRGs, care plans, and nursing diagnoses—when used separately, has a specific role in the health care delivery system. DRGs quantify medical care and its cost, care plans facilitate the evaluation of patients' responses to the therapeutic regimen, and nursing diagnoses serve as a prescription for the nursing care rendered.

The combination of a nursing care plan based on nursing diagnoses and linked to DRGs gives the professional nurse the most concrete instrument for quantifying nursing to date. **Nursing Diagnosis Care Plans** provides us with that instrument.

I believe this text will become required reading for all nurses who wish to survive in this era of cost containment, where the value of one's contribution to the health care delivery system must be demonstrable and measurable.

For providing us with a usable, workable, simple guide to quantify nursing as a profession and for their vision, timeliness, and clarity of purpose, we owe a debt of gratitude to the authors.

Rosalinda Haddon, RN, MA
Assistant Director
Newark Beth Israel Medical Center
Newark, New Jersey

Preface   All health care professionals are striving to upgrade patient care. Nurses are particularly concerned with providing health care to ever-increasing patient populations without sacrificing individualized care. This requires careful planning of nursing interventions for each patient, a process that is assisted and structured by the nursing care plan. During audits, it is often said, "If it isn't in the care plan, it isn't being done." Nursing care plans allow continuity and coordination of patient care; they help nurses set priorities and evaluate patient response, and they are vital in documenting and justifying the need for service variations.

In the present era, nurses in acute care facilities are assuming more direct responsibility for total patient care. The value and use of nursing diagnosis is increasingly obvious to the authors and to nursing colleagues; all have repeatedly bemoaned the lack of an accepted nomenclature. The impetus to write this book stems from personal frustration at the lack of standardization in nursing care plans, at the difficulty associating nursing diagnoses with the plan of care, and at not knowing how to correctly document nursing care.

Nursing care plans are the key to professional nursing care and *must* be written for specific nursing diagnoses to document the care needed, the care given, and the patient responses. This book is a tool with suggested guidelines to make this job easier.

Velma C. Frey
Christine Hockett
Gerri Moist

Acknowledgments

To M. Shelley Young, RN, PhD, whose interest and guidance kept us going in the right direction

To Sandra Stone, RN, MS, whose encouragement and experience expanded our horizon

To Connie Harrison, RN, who willingly supplied information

To Betty M. Hockett, freelance writer, who shared her adventures in writing and showed us a dream could become a reality

To Glenna C. Young, for her great patience in doing the typing

To all our colleagues who voiced their frustration with writing nursing care plans.

Contents

Introduction

All nurses are aware of the importance of written documentation of the care they provide, but not all are familiar with the standard language that has come into use in recent years. Standardization is the key to documentation for legal and third-party payment purposes, and to effective communication between all health care providers.

Toward that end, the National Group for the Classification of Nursing Diagnoses was formed in 1973. Its seven conferences to date have resulted in over 50 standard nursing diagnoses, diagnoses with which many nurses still struggle when formulating their everyday care plans. This book provides general guidelines to help incorporate nursing diagnoses into patient care plans.

The authors supplement the list of nursing diagnoses accepted at the national conferences with realistic assessments, interventions, and outcome criteria for each diagnosis. A suggested format for utilizing this information is also included.

We do not pretend to have included all possible information. The focus of this book is broad, not slanted toward any specialized nursing area but rather toward general patient care. This handbook is designed to help *all* nursing readers, whether students or practicing members of the health care team, use the diagnostic material to begin formulating plans for individualized nursing care. A suggested method for using this reference follows.

When a patient is admitted, perform standard assessment and identify areas of nursing focus. Select the applicable nursing diagnoses, assessments, interventions, evaluation criteria, and expected outcomes. Enter them on the nursing care plan form, along with any additional relevant ideas. Next, use the hospital's "Diagnosis Related Groups" reference to determine appropriate target dates for cited outcomes. Finally, document all assessments and treatments, along with the patient's responses, in the proper record and update it as the patient's condition warrants. The patient's chart must be consistent with the care plan.

To individualize nursing care plans, it is imperative that the nurse take into account the acuity of the patient's condition, as well as priorities and past experiences. Only then can appropriate interventions be chosen, a proper timetable (i.e., frequency of intervention and limits for evaluation) assigned and realistic goals set. Spelling out the reactions and the times assigned to them ensures continuity of care for individual needs—the vital essence of nursing.

ACTIVITY INTOLERANCE, ACTUAL OR POTENTIAL

Nursing Diagnosis

Potential Clinical Findings

History of activity intolerance
Shortness of breath with activity
Cardiac or respiratory problems
Fatigue with activity
Orthostatic hypotension
Pain
Limited muscle and bone movement
Obesity
Decreased motivation in social activities and in ADL

Expected Outcomes

- The patient will achieve/maintain a level of activity tolerance for self-care (specify individual level).
- The patient will develop/maintain a functional level of social activity (specify level).
- The patient will develop/maintain maximal independent activity (specify individual level).

Interventions

- Assess the source, extent, and implications of the impairment (e.g., acute versus chronic, life-style changes).
- Do history and physical assessment.
- Evaluate activity/rest pattern and level of activity.
- Monitor and document

  - vital signs with activity
  - complaints of fatigue, shortness of breath, muscle pain and fatigue, and range of motion with varied activities
  - ECG changes
  - x-ray reports

- Place in position of comfort; reposition at least every 2 hours.

- Assist with ADL as necessary.
- Encourage adequate rest periods; provide periods of rest during care.
- Anticipate needs (avoids anxiety).
- Monitor lab results and report significant values
    - ABGs
    - CBC
    - diff
    - sed rate
    - chem profile
    - electrolyte levels
    - UA
- Provide appropriate adaptive equipment (e.g., splints, walkers, elevated toilet seat).
- Monitor effects of prescribed medications.
- Teach patient to recognize signs of fatigue and intolerance and to rest accordingly.
- Contract with patient to maintain regular program of physical activity to gradually increase tolerance (specify contract made).
- Monitor vital signs with activity.
- Instruct patient about potential for activity intolerance caused by existing problems (specify).
- Allow adequate time for completion of tasks.
- Give support as needed and encourage patient to perform activities as tolerated.
- Provide opportunity for and promote patient interaction with others.
- Praise all accomplishments and gains that patient makes.
- Include family in all instructions regarding extent of the impairment and participation in selected interven-

tions (specify instruction and interventions).
- Teach patient about medications and the importance of maintaining prescribed regimen.

Outcome Criteria

- The patient adequately performs specified activities within tolerance as evidenced by stable vital signs, no undue fatigue, weakness, or dyspnea.
- The patient shows increased interaction with others.

Potentially Related Nursing Diagnoses

Breathing pattern, ineffective
Cardiac output, alteration in: decreased
Comfort, alteration in: pain
Mobility, impaired physical
Self-care deficit (specify level)
Tissue perfusion, alteration in

Diagnosis Related Groups

- Diseases and Disorders of the Nervous System (e.g., spinal disorders and injuries, degenerative nervous system disorders)
- Diseases and Disorders of the Ear, Nose, and Throat (e.g., disequilibrium, neurologic eye disorders)
- Diseases and Disorders of the Respiratory System (e.g., pulmonary embolism, pulmonary edema, and respiratory failure)
- Diseases and Disorders of the Circulatory System (e.g., coronary bypass, peripheral vascular disorders)

- Diseases and Disorders of the Digestive System (e.g., GI, hemorrhage, digestive malignancy)
- Diseases and Disorders of the Musculoskeletal System and Connective Tissues (e.g., tendonitis, myositis and bursitis, amputations)

Nursing Diagnosis

AIRWAY CLEARANCE, INEFFECTIVE

Potential Clinical Findings

Purulent sputum
Rales, rhonchi
Choking sensation
Inspiratory/expiratory wheezing
Shortness of breath, feelings of air hunger
Inability to speak
Use of ancillary breathing muscles
Presence of foreign bodies in respiratory tract
Stridor
Unequal breath sounds
Edema in respiratory tract
Rapid, labored respirations
Chest pain with or without splinting
Anxiety
Frequent cough

Expected Outcomes

- The patient will maintain a patent airway.
- The patient will breathe at an even and unlabored rate.
- The patient's lungs will be clear to auscultation.

Interventions

- Evaluate air exchange (e.g., skin color, breath sounds, complaints of dyspnea, anxiety).
- Provide and maintain a patent airway (e.g., remove foreign objects, reposition, place artificial airway, institute emergency protocol for respiratory arrest).
- Evaluate effectiveness of prescribed oxygen and medications.
- Elevate head of bed until patient breathes more easily.

- Insert IV if indicated.
- Complete a chest assessment (including inspection, auscultation, and percussion).
- Monitor

  - vital signs
  - ECG changes
  - respiration characteristics (rate, depth, etc.)
  - sputum characteristics (consistency, color, amount, etc.)
  - x-ray reports

- Suction as needed; record number of times, color, and consistency of secretions.
- Monitor lab results and report significant values

  - ABGs
  - CBC
  - diff
  - sed rate
  - electrolytes
  - chem profile
  - theophylline level
  - sputum gram stain, C&S
  - sputum AFB
  - UA

- Monitor effectiveness of prescribed respiratory treatments.
- Minimize environmental stress (e.g., limited interruptions, quiet room).
- Demonstrate and teach adaptive breathing methods (e.g., pursed lip, rebreathing through paper bag, slow and deliberate respiratory rate).
- Turn patient, encourage coughing and deep breathing if indicated, at least every 2 hours and as necessary.
- Teach proper disposal of secretions.

- Ensure a cool, moist airflow in the room to minimize airborn irritants, decrease body oxygen requirements, and support patient's psychologic sense of adequate air flow.
- Use lemon juice, warm drinks, etc., to aid expectoration of secretions.
- Work with patient to identify airway irritants and ways to avoid them.
- Teach patient signs and symptoms of respiratory infection (e.g., fever, chills, shortness of breath, sputum changes) and what to do when these appear.
- Teach patient about medications and the importance of maintaining prescribed regimen.

Outcome Criteria

The patient aerates lungs adequately as evidenced by clear breath sounds; even, unlabored respirations; verbalization of increased ease in breathing.

Potentially Related Nursing Diagnoses

Activity intolerance
Fluid volume, alteration in: excess
Fluid volume deficit, actual or potential
Gas exchange, impaired

Diagnosis Related Groups

- Diseases and Disorders of the Nervous System (e.g., stupor and coma, multiple sclerosis, and cerebellar ataxia)
- Diseases and Disorders of the Ear, Nose, and Throat (e.g., major head and neck procedures, epiglottis)

- Diseases and Disorders of the Respiratory System (e.g., bronchitis and asthma, major chest trauma)
- Diseases and Disorders of the Circulatory System (e.g., heart failure and shock, major reconstructive vascular procedures)

ANXIETY

Mild level

- broad perceptual field
- ability to take in multiple stimuli
- relaxed muscle and facial tension
- feelings of safety and comfort

Moderate level

- narrowed perceptual field
- ability to solve problems
- optimal level for learning
- increased alertness and tension
- feelings of challenge and a need to handle situation

Severe level

- greatly reduced perceptual field
- distorted time sense
- survival response (fight or flight)
- feelings of increasing threat
- increased physical activity that is purposeless
- selective inattention
- personal space is extended

Panic level

- closed perceptual field (tunnel vision)
- random thoughts, impaired thinking
- unable to solve problems, scattered
- poor motor coordination
- increased physiologic arousal
- feelings of helplessness, anger, dread, terror
- may strike out or withdraw
- pressured speech, blocked speech
- unable to function

Other physiologic and psychologic manifestations seen in severe panic levels

- agitation
- apprehension
- cold, pale skin
- diaphoresis
- diarrhea
- dread
- dry mouth
- elevated BP
- escalated speech
- feeling of doom
- flighty ideas
- indecisiveness
- irritability
- muscle tension
- nausea
- nervousness
- palpitations
- panic
- poor immediate recall of number series
- repetitive motions
- tachycardia
- tachypnea
- tearfulness
- tremors
- urinary frequency

Expected Outcomes

- The patient will reduce anxiety to a mild-moderate level.
- The patient will achieve or maintain a functional status.

Interventions

- Identify the patient's level of anxiety.
- Monitor physiologic, psychologic, and cognitive functioning (see Potential Clinical Findings).
- Identify stressors and precipitating factors.
- Monitor lab results and report significant values (rule out organic etiology)

    – ABGs
    – CBC
    – electrolytes
    – serum drug screen

Mild-Moderate level

- Realize that this is an optimal level for learning and utilize the opportunity to educate patient about treatments, procedures, and relaxation techniques.

- Keep anxiety from escalating by providing consistent care and brief, factual information as needed.
- Identify alleviating factors that can be instituted to prevent anxiety from increasing.
- Provide meaningful diversional activities.
- Give valid reassurance and reinforce positive behaviors.
- Identify and promote proven effective coping mechanisms.
- Teach and encourage use of stress management techniques.
- Promote patient participation in problem solving as appropriate.

Severe-Panic level

- Provide a quiet atmosphere, reduce external stimuli.
- Speak simply and directly, using a calm, modulated voice.
- Avoid contributing to the patient's maladaptive behavior (specify behavior, e.g., screaming, blaming others, manipulating staff); maintain firm, consistent approach with patient.
- Stay with patient and listen therapeutically; avoid asking "why" questions, it raises anxiety.
- Repeat statements as necessary. Allow patient to set pace for interaction.
- Encourage patient to use slow, deep breathing; use relaxation techniques.
- Encourage patient to verbalize feelings (e.g., "What are you feeling right now?").
- Elicit descriptions of stressful events that precipitated the anxiety (e.g., "Where were you? Who was there? What did you say?").

- Recognize signs of increasing anxiety and the need for physical release of energy (e.g., walking, running, pounding a punching bag, yelling provide outlets for anxiety).
- Allow ample personal space; do not touch the patient unless asked or patient is in need of restraining.
- Decrease stimuli by avoiding detailed explanations. Communicate in short, simple, and direct statements.
- Determine with the patient what new or modified behaviors would be more effective in dealing with anxiety.
- Lend perspective about the situation to widen the perceptual field and open up "tunnel vision."
- Provide self-help measures: bath, exercises, back rub, warm milk, or wine.
- Be aware that anxiety is contagious and monitor your own reactions. Use deep breathing, quiet pauses, to maintain equilibrium.
- Evaluate the effect of prescribed medications (antianxiety) and treatments.

Outcome Criteria

- The patient has mild-moderate anxiety as evidenced by ability to concentrate, verbalization of precipitating factors, relaxed affect.
- The patient focuses on and completes tasks at hand.
- The patient understands the origins of the anxiety and has new ways to deal with it.

Potentially Related Nursing Diagnoses All diagnoses

Diagnosis Related Groups Potentially applicable within all diagnosis related groups

Nursing Diagnosis

BOWEL ELIMINATION, ALTERATION IN: CONSTIPATION

Potential Clinical Findings

Abdomen distended, firm
Decreased bowel tones
Elderly
Poor diet
Decreased frequency of elimination
Painful elimination
Feeling of abdominal fullness
Nausea and vomiting
Hard, dry stool
High-pitched bowel sounds
Signs of dehydration

Expected Outcomes

- The patient will eliminate soft-formed stool at regular intervals.
- The patient will verbalize an increase in comfort.

Interventions

- Do abdominal assessment (including inspection, auscultation, percussion, and palpation in that order).
- Complete a digital exam unless otherwise indicated.
- Remove any impaction palpable on digital exam.
- Assess patient's own remedies for constipation.
- Evaluate medications received and their effects.
- Monitor

  - abdominal characteristics (distention, firmness, masses, and tenderness)
  - nausea and vomiting
  - bowel sounds in all four quadrants
  - orthostatic vital signs (rule out shock status secondary to bowel

perforation, etc., and as indicator of fluid balance)
- intake and output
- stool characteristics (color, consistency, frequency, and amount)
- daily weights
- lab results and report significant values

* CBC
* chem profile
* electrolytes
* stool occult blood

- diagnostic procedure reports

• Maintain npo as ordered (constipation can be a symptom of bowel obstruction).
• Insert and maintain nasogastric tube as ordered.
• Administer laxative of choice, stool softener, bulk agent, or enema as ordered; monitor effects.
• Provide for regular, uninterrupted elimination time.
• Force fluids unless otherwise indicated (specify amount).
• Provide a high-fiber diet unless otherwise indicated.
• Offer prune juice with breakfast.
• Promote activity as tolerated (e.g., walking, rocking in chair, stretching and relaxing while lying in bed).
• Teach patient about medications and the importance of maintaining prescribed regimen.

Outcome Criteria

• The patient has improved bowel function as evidenced by regular elimination of soft-formed stool.
• The patient reports increased comfort.

Potentially Related Nursing Diagnoses

Comfort, alteration in: pain
Fear
Fluid volume deficit, actual or potential
Knowledge deficit (specify)
Nutrition, alteration in: less than body requirements

Diagnosis Related Groups

- Diseases and Disorders of the Nervous System (e.g., spinal disorders and injuries; cranial and peripheral nerve disorders)
- Diseases and Disorders of the Circulatory System (e.g., cardiac dysrhythmias, angina pectoris)
- Diseases and Disorders of the Respiratory System (e.g., chronic obstructive pulmonary disease; interstitial lung disease)
- Diseases and Disorders of the Digestive System (e.g., GI obstruction, digestive system procedures)

BOWEL ELIMINATION, ALTERATION IN: DIARRHEA

Nursing Diagnosis

Potential Clinical Findings

Increased frequency of liquid stools
Scattered stools
Tarry, foamy, bloody stools
Abdominal cramping and pain
Weakness
Irritated, reddened anus
Anal fissures
Fever
Malaise
Hyperactive bowel sounds
Dry oral membranes
Decreased skin turgor

Expected Outcomes

- The patient will eliminate soft-formed stool at regular intervals.
- The patient will verbalize increased comfort.

Interventions

- Do abdominal assessment (including inspection, auscultation, percussion, and palpation).
- Evaluate history for acute versus chronic diarrhea.
- Complete a digital exam unless otherwise indicated.
- Assess history of recent travel and diet.
- Evaluate effects of patient's medications.
- Maintain enteric isolation until otherwise indicated.
- Provide meticulous perineal care after each elimination; give sitz baths as ordered.
- Monitor lab results and report significant values

- CBC
- chem profile
- electrolytes
- stool C&S
- ova and parasites
- occult blood

• Monitor and document

- daily weight
- intake and output
- stool consistency, color, frequency
- diagnostic procedure reports (e.g., x-ray, sigmoidoscopy)

• Monitor IV for patency and flow; maintain site.
• Replace fluid loss per daily requirements.
• Maintain npo as ordered.
• Evaluate effects of prescribed medications.
• Provide bulk or low-residue diet when indicated.
• Reduce environmental stress.
• Encourage patient to express own feelings and fears verbally; use leading statements and questions to allow patient opportunity to discuss emotional stress (e.g., "You sound angry;" "How do you feel right now?").
• Provide nutritional instruction as indicated.
• Teach patient about medications and importance of maintaining prescribed regimen.

Outcome Criteria

• The patient eliminates soft-formed stool regularly.
• The patient verbalizes increased comfort (e.g.., decreased abdominal cramping and pain).

Potentially Related Nursing Diagnoses

Comfort, alteration in: pain
Fear
Fluid volume deficit, actual or potential
Nutrition, alteration in: less than body requirements
Self-care deficit (specify level)
Self-concept, disturbance in
Skin integrity, impairment of: potential
Sleep pattern disturbance

Diagnosis Related Groups

- Diseases and Disorders of the Digestive System (e.g., inflammatory bowel disease, gastroenteritis)
- Diseases and Disorders of the Hepatobiliary System and Pancreas (e.g., cirrhosis and alcoholic hepatitis, malignancy of hepatobiliary system and pancreas)
- Endocrine, Nutritional, and Metabolic Diseases and Disorders (e.g., hyperthyroidism, surgical procedures for obesity)
- Newborns and other Neonates with Conditions Originating in the Perinatal Period (e.g., neonate extreme immaturity, neonatal sepsis)
- Infectious and Parasitic Diseases (e.g., allergic reactions, toxic effects of drugs)

BOWEL ELIMINATION, ALTERATION IN: INCONTINENCE

Nursing Diagnosis

Potential Clinical Findings

Involuntary stooling
Irritated, reddened anus
Perineal skin breakdown
Neurologic deficits
Decreased anal sphincter tone
Impaired mobility
Excessive bowel preparations for diagnostic/surgical procedures

Expected Outcomes

- The patient will be clean and dry with skin intact.
- The patient will participate in establishing a regular bowel routine.

Interventions

- Do abdominal assessment (including inspection, auscultation, percussion, and palpation).
- Perform a digital exam assessing for sphincter tone and sensation.
- Assess patient's awareness of stool incontinency.
- Provide

  - soft linen and padding that allow air to circulate to the skin
  - meticulous perineal hygiene after each elimination
  - sitz baths as ordered

- Turn and reposition at least every 2 hours.
- Monitor and chart

  - frequency of stooling
  - stool characteristics
  - restlessness
  - diagnostic procedure reports

- Monitor lab results and report significant values

  - CBC
  - electrolytes
  - stool C&S, occult blood

- Begin to establish regular bowel routine (i.e., place patient on commode or bedpan after meals or at consistent intervals); involve care givers and patient when instructing on bowel regimen.
- Evaluate effectiveness of rectal tube, if ordered.
- Evaluate effects of prescribed medications.
- Provide honest reassurance, especially if condition is temporary.
- Instruct patient and care givers on proper diet and exercise routines.
- Have patient and/or care givers return demonstrate bowel regimen and exercise routines.
- Teach patient/family about required medications and the importance of maintaining prescribed regimen.

Outcome Criteria

- The patient maintains skin integrity as evidenced by clean, dry, and intact skin.
- The patient participates in establishing a regular bowel regimen (e.g., consistently requests bedpan, commode, etc., at established intervals; follows diet and medication regimen; utilizes digital stimulation).

Potentially Related Nursing Diagnoses

Comfort, alteration in: pain
Home maintenance management, impaired
Knowledge deficit (specify)

Powerlessness
Self-care deficit (specify level)

**Diagnosis
Related Groups**

- Diseases and Disorders of the Nervous System (e.g., nervous system neoplasms, degenerative nervous system disorders)
- Diseases and Disorders of the Digestive System (e.g., minor small and large bowel procedures, anal procedures)

Nursing Diagnosis

BREATHING PATTERN, INEFFECTIVE

Potential Clinical Findings

Nasal flaring
Chest retractions
Inspiratory/expiratory wheezing
Rales, rhonchi
Pain
Activity intolerance
Rapid, shallow respirations
Irregular respirations
Tachycardia
Fever
Dry mucous membranes
Feeling of air hunger
Numbness and tingling of extremities

Expected Outcomes

- The patient will verbalize an increase in comfort.
- The patient will breathe at an even and unlabored rate.
- The patient's lungs will be clear to auscultation.

Interventions

- Do chest assessment (including inspection, auscultation, and percussion).
- Evaluate patient's sensorium and level of fatigue.
- Identify if condition is acute or chronic.
- Position in orthopneic position or position of comfort.
- Monitor and document

  - respiration characteristics (e.g., rate, depth)
  - vital signs
  - breath sounds
  - skin color and turgor
  - level of comfort

- ECGs
- x-ray reports
- intake and output
- daily weights

- Monitor lab results and report significant values

  - CBC
  - ABGs
  - chem profile
  - electrolytes
  - PT
  - PTT
  - theophylline level if indicated
  - UA
  - sputum C&S

- Evaluate effects of prescribed oxygen, medications.
- Demonstrate and teach adaptive breathing methods (e.g., pursed lip, rebreathing through paper bag, slow deliberate respirations).
- Evaluate effects of prescribed respiratory treatments.
- Provide or restrict fluids as condition indicates (specify amounts).
- Plan nursing care to include rest periods, quiet time.
- Reduce environmental stress (e.g., approach patient in a calm manner, provide nonsmoking area, maintain quiet atmosphere).
- Provide a cool room with air circulation and controlled humidity.
- Work with patient to identify precipitating factors of ineffective breathing patterns and ways to avoid them.
- Teach patient the importance of balancing activity and rest periods.
- Teach patient signs and symptoms of respiratory infection (e.g., fever,

change in sputum, increased cough), and what to do when they occur.

- Teach patient about prescribed medications and the importance of maintaining regimen.

Outcome Criteria

- The patient is well oxygenated as evidenced by even and unlabored respirations, increased aeration throughout the lungs, no chest retractions, clear breath sounds, pink nailbeds, no numbness or tingling of extremities.
- The patient's affect is relaxed; the patient states it is now easier to breathe.

Potentially Related Nursing Diagnoses

Activity intolerance, actual or potential
Airway clearance, ineffective
Cardiac output, alteration in: decreased
Comfort, alteration in: pain
Fluid volume, alteration in: excess
Gas exchange, impaired

Diagnosis Related Groups

- Diseases and Disorders of the Nervous System (e.g., seizures, traumatic stupor and coma)
- Diseases and Disorders of the Ear, Nose, and Throat (e.g., major head and neck procedures, nose and throat malignancy)
- Diseases and Disorders of the Respiratory System (e.g., respiratory infections and inflammations, chest trauma)
- Diseases and Disorders of the Circulatory System (e.g., major reconstructive vascular procedures, heart failure and shock)

CARDIAC OUTPUT, ALTERATION IN: DECREASED

Nursing Diagnosis

Potential Clinical Findings

Fatigue
Poor tissue perfusion
Dysrhythmias
Muffled heart sounds
Edema
Weight gain
Anxiety
Rales
Tachypnea
Altered mental status
Tachycardia
Bradycardia

Expected Outcomes

- The patient will achieve adequate cardiac output.
- The patient will be able to identify signs and symptoms of decreasing cardiac output.

Interventions

- Do circulatory and respiratory assessment.
- Evaluate effects of prescribed oxygen, medications.
- Monitor and document

  - vital signs
  - ECGs
  - systemic perfusion (color and temperature of extremities and capillary refill)
  - venous engorgement
  - intake and output
  - fatigue
  - daily weight
  - breath sounds
  - edema (check for dependent and sacral edema)

- mental status
- diagnostic procedure reports

- Monitor lab results and report significant values
  - ABGs
  - CBC
  - chem profile
  - electrolytes
  - PT
  - PTT
- Place in position of comfort.
- Reposition patient every 2 hours and elevate extremities as indicated by edema.
- Administer care and regulate the environment to decrease the cardiac workload (e.g., cool temperature, quiet surroundings, calm manner, assist patient with ADL).
- Maintain and/or titrate
  - IVs
  - hemodynamic pressure lines
  - cardiac output measurements as indicated
- Explain all diagnostic tests and procedures.
- Instruct about importance of sodium-restricted diet unless otherwise indicated.
- Teach patient about signs and symptoms of decreasing cardiac output (e.g., edema and weight gain, fatigue, shortness of breath).
- Teach patient about prescribed medications and the importance of maintaining regimen.

Outcome Criteria

- The patient has adequate cardiac output as evidenced by stable vital signs, reduced venous engorgement and

edema, warm extremities, adequate capillary refill, appropriate orientation.
- The patient can identify signs and symptoms of decreasing cardiac output (specify those taught).

Potentially Related Nursing Diagnoses

Activity intolerance, actual or potential
Fear
Home maintenance management, impaired
Knowledge deficit (specify)
Mobility, impaired physical
Sexual dysfunction

Diagnosis Related Groups

- Diseases and Disorders of the Circulatory System (e.g., heart failure and shock, circulatory disorders with AMI)
- Diseases and Disorders of the Respiratory System (e.g., pulmonary edema, major chest trauma)

Nursing Diagnosis

COMFORT, ALTERATION IN: PAIN

Potential Clinical Findings

Verbalization of pain
Tense affect
Guarded movement
Splinting
Nausea and vomiting
Fatigue
Depression
Tachycardia
Tachypnea
Inflammation
Erythema
Swollen joints

Expected Outcomes

The patient will experience an increase in comfort.

Interventions

- Do assessment to determine systems involved.
- Evaluate if acute or chronic pain.
- Assess and document
  - pain characteristics (location, intensity, frequency, duration, aggravating and alleviating factors)
  - patient behaviors (facial affect, posture, movement, voice tone, speech, activity)
  - diagnostic procedure data
- Monitor lab results and report significant values
  - CBC
  - sed rate
  - chem profile
  - electrolytes
  - UA
- Evaluate effects of prescribed medications.

- Encourage diversional activities (e.g., conversation, television, reading, performance of tasks).
- Promote relaxation (e.g., provide a quiet atmosphere, give back rub, place in position of comfort).
- Utilize relaxation techniques; supplement with tape recordings.
- Utilize heat and/or cold therapy to affected area unless otherwise indicated.
- Explore with patient what needs pain might be meeting and assist in exploring rational alternatives; help the patient to identify consequences of each alternative.
- Avoid encouraging maladaptive behavior (e.g., do not pay more attention to patient only when complaining of pain).
- Teach patient about prescribed medications and the importance of maintaining regimen.

Outcome Criteria

The patient experiences pain control as evidenced by

- verbalization of increased comfort
- 24-hour abstention from parenteral pain medication
- appropriate patient interaction with staff, visitors, other patients
- increased ease of movement.

Potentially Related Nursing Diagnoses

Activity intolerance, actual or potential
Coping, ineffective individual
Diversional activity, deficit
Fear
Nutrition, alteration in: less than body requirements

Oral mucous membrane, alteration in
Self-concept, disturbance in
Sleep pattern disturbance
Spiritual distress

Diagnosis Related Groups   Potentially applicable within all diagnosis related groups

COMMUNICATION, IMPAIRED: VERBAL

Nursing Diagnosis

Potential Clinical Findings

Aphasia (motor/sensory)
Anxiety
Foreign language barrier
Coma
Fear
Hard of hearing/deafness
Depression
Tracheostomy
Endotracheal tube in place
Post-neck surgery
Laryngectomy

Expected Outcomes

The patient will display adequate bilateral communication skills.

Interventions

- Assess the source and extent of impairment (acute versus chronic).
- Evaluate the patient's current method and level of communication.
- Utilize nonverbal communication techniques
  - call system (e.g., quad or touch light)
  - eye blinking, tongue movement (simple movements for yes and no)
  - written material (Zygo board, cue cards, etc.)
  - hand gestures
  - writing supplies
- Ask one question at a time; repeat as necessary, allowing adequate time for each response.
- Use short simple sentences; match patient's level of understanding.
- Explain all procedures and tasks, even when patient is unable to respond.

- Anticipate patient's needs.
- Utilize appropriate assistive devices (e.g., hearing aids, voice box).
- Speak clearly and at an appropriate volume; project directly to the patient, maintaining direct eye contact.
- Use interpreters when available (e.g., foreign language, sign language, individual adapted language).
- Validate information with the patient (e.g., "I understood you to say . . . Is that correct?").

Outcome Criteria

The patient communicates adequately as evidenced by appropriate responses to communications from others, relaxed facial affect, expressed satisfaction with methods of communication, expression of needs and wants.

Potentially Related Nursing Diagnoses

Anxiety
Coping, ineffective individual/family
Family process, alteration in
Fear
Grieving, anticipatory
Oral mucous membrane, alteration in
Self-concept, disturbance in

Diagnosis Related Groups

- Diseases and Disorders of the Nervous System (e.g., craniotomy, degenerative nervous system disorders)
- Diseases and Disorders of the Ear, Nose, and Throat (e.g., ear, nose, throat malignancy; miscellaneous ear, nose, throat procedures)

- Diseases and Disorders of the Respiratory System (e.g., pulmonary failure and respiratory failure, major chest procedures)
- Diseases and Disorders of the Circulatory System (e.g., cardiothoracic procedures, cardiac arrest)

COPING, FAMILY: POTENTIAL FOR GROWTH

Nursing Diagnosis

**Potential
Clinical Findings**

Family involved in adapting to patient's illness
Family exhibits willingness to learn
Family expresses desire to overcome the crisis and move forward
Effective family communication
Successful completion of previous stages of development
Effectively provide emotional support for one another

**Expected
Outcomes**

- The family will be able to demonstrate effective utilization of coping skills (specify desired skills, e.g., planning alternatives, utilizing outside resources).
- The family members will recognize how the crisis/illness has enhanced growth.

Interventions

- Assess strengths and weaknesses of the family group and individual members.
- Assess each member's developmental stage as well as that of the family as a unit.
- Identify individual members' coping skills.
- Identify family resources

    - satisfaction and relationships
    - how decisions are made and by whom
    - hierarchy (who sets limits/discipline, who helps with what tasks)
    - marital stability
    - communication patterns
    - relationship with extended family

- religious beliefs and practices
- ability to organize after a crisis
- adaptation to organization and management of daily schedule changes since diagnosis
- sacrifices necessary for family function and feelings regarding sacrifices
- expectations of each member
- financial, educational, and cultural status
- basic physical resources (home, health care, crisis prevention, equipment needs, clothing and food)

- Encourage family to

    - maximize its strengths (in communication, respect, cooperation, demonstrating affection, etc.)
    - utilize effective, reality-oriented coping skills and resources
    - successfully complete current developmental tasks
    - develop assertive, effective communication patterns

- Provide valid reassurance (correct misinformation, offer only factual information, be sincere).
- Promote outside interests.
- Provide opportunities for family to explore and test new coping skills (e.g., problem solving, prioritizing, planning alternatives).
- Listen therapeutically (i.e., provide opportunity for family members to verbalize feelings and needs, encourage use of "I" messages to state feelings and needs).
- Encourage family members to continue participation in outside interest

(e.g., hobbies, sports, crafts, occupations).
- Offer information about support groups and outside agencies of mutual interest.

Outcome Criteria

- Family demonstrates effective utilization of coping skills as evidenced by continuation through developmental tasks and statements of satisfaction with knowledge gained for adapting (specify knowledge gained).
- Family members recognize enhanced growth as evidenced by statements of increased closeness, expressions of future plans, and verbal acknowledgement of change.

Potentially Related Nursing Diagnoses

Coping, ineffective individual/family
Family process, alteration in
Knowledge deficit (specify)

Diagnosis Related Groups

Potentially applicable within all diagnosis related groups

COPING, INEFFECTIVE FAMILY: COMPROMISED

Nursing Diagnosis

Potential Clinical Findings

Temporary family disorganization
Prolonged illness exhausting significant others
Knowledge deficit about illness
Unrealistic expectations of patient's wants and needs
Overprotective significant others
Inadequate knowledge base regarding support of ill family member
A usually supportive primary person becomes nonsupportive

Expected Outcomes

Family members will adequately and effectively provide the support and encouragement necessary for the patient to meet own wants and needs.

Interventions

- Work with family to identify stressors to ineffective coping.
- Assess strengths and weaknesses in family's ability to problem solve (e.g., individual characteristics, developmental stages).
- Provide opportunities for the family to explore and test problem-solving skills.
- Explore past experiences and support systems, family values and goals.
- Identify family resources

  - satisfaction with relationships
  - how decisions are made and by whom
  - hierarchy (who sets limits/discipline, who helps with what tasks)
  - marital stability
  - communication patterns
  - relationship with extended family

- religious beliefs and practices
- ability to organize after a crisis
- adaptation to organization and management of daily schedule change since diagnosis
  sacrifices necessary for family function and feelings regarding sacrifices
- expectations of each member
- financial, educational, and cultural status
- basic physical resources (home, health care, crisis prevention, equipment needs, clothing and food)

- Encourage family mobilization and use of internal and external resources (specify resources available to family).
- Explore family functions in community and leisure activities.
- Encourage family members to continue participation in outside interests.
- Evaluate family's decision making abilities.
- Provide opportunity for family to explore alternatives in decision making; teach family to explore consequences of each alternative.
- Teach family to effectively use communication skills.
- Provide opportunity for family to utilize new communication skills (e.g., role playing, family meetings).
- Encourage family members to accept feeling statements as valid.
- Listen therapeutically (e.g., encourage use of "I" statements to state feelings and needs).

- Help family members focus on their own strengths, potential.
- Identify other situational or developmental crisis or underlying problems that may contribute to family's inability to support patient.
- Determine chronic and long-term situations (length of illness, disability, low finances) that are undermining family's reserves.
- Discuss with family the role of the patient and how illness has altered family organization and functioning.
- Discuss with family the underlying reasons for patient's behaviors to assist them to accept and support the patient during the illness.
- Sort out the various problems and help patient and family recognize who is responsible for the resolutions.

Outcome Criteria

- Family members adequately and effectively assist patient to meet own wants and needs as evidenced by their involvement with discharge planning, participation in daily patient care, and verbalization of confidence to cope with the situation (specify).
- Patient verbalizes satisfaction that family helps to meet wants and needs.

Potentially Related Nursing Diagnoses

Family process, alteration in
Grieving, anticipatory
Knowledge deficit (specify)
Parenting, alteration in: actual or potential

Diagnosis Related Groups Potentially applicable within all diagnosis related groups

COPING, INEFFECTIVE FAMILY: DISABLING

Nursing Diagnosis

Potential Clinical Findings

Neglect of patient's needs
Prolonged overconcern for patient
Abuse, abandonment
Unrealistic expectations
Family unit dissolving
Anger, aggression
Maladaptive coping behaviors detrimental to welfare of the patient
Depression, agitation, hostility
Intolerance of illness behaviors
Ambivalent family relationships
Distortion of reality of patient's health problem (denial)

Expected Outcomes

The family will exhibit behaviors that enable members to effectively adapt to the current situation.

Interventions

- Work with family to assess the patient's physical and emotional needs.
- Assess family's emotional needs, coping skills, strengths and weaknesses in family relationships, family's insight into the current problem(s).
- Help family recognize disabling condition(s).
- Identify family resources

  - satisfaction with relationships
  - how decisions are made and by whom
  - hierarchy (who sets limits/discipline, who helps with what tasks)
  - marital stability
  - communication patterns
  - relationship with extended family
  - religious beliefs and practices
  - ability to organize after a crisis

- adaptation to organization and management of daily schedule changes since diagnosis
- sacrifices necessary for family function; feelings regarding sacrifices
- expectations of each member
- financial, educational, and cultural status
- basic physical resources (home, health care, crisis prevention, equipment needs, clothing, food)

- Encourage family mobilization and use of internal and external resources (specify available resources).
- Listen therapeutically (e.g., encourage use of "I" statements to state feelings and needs, provide opportunity for family members to verbalize their feelings and needs).
- Encourage family members to accept feeling statements as valid.
- Teach family to effectively use communication skills.
- Provide opportunity for family to practice new communication skills.
- Assess learning readiness and begin teaching about specific disability and management of affected member(s).
- Encourage family to negotiate and compromise regarding necessary sacrifices and duties.
- Provide opportunity for family members to role play use of negotiation and compromise.
- Help family members to set concrete goals consistent with their values and needs.
- Encourage family involvement in outside interests.

- Offer information about support groups and outside agencies of mutual interest.
- Obtain consults from other members of the health care team as indicated (specify members consulted).
- Assess pre-illness status of the family (interactions, behaviors, roles).
- Identify family's behavioral responses to the patient (e.g., anger, withdrawal, blaming).
- Establish rapport with family and determine their readiness to deal with the situation.
- Provide ongoing and accurate information to patient and family; give brief, simple explanations about equipment and procedures.
- Act as a liaison between patient, family, and hospital staff; demonstrate clear communication techniques in interactions with family.
- Give feedback to family on how their coping strategies are not helping them deal with the situation; explore alternative behaviors.
- Give support and positive reinforcement to family when they demonstrate constructive coping and new attitudes.

Outcome Criteria

The family exhibits behaviors of effective coping with current situation as evidenced by use of negotiation and compromise, family involvement in discharge planning, verbalization of confidence in coping with the situation (specify).

Potentially Related Nursing Diagnoses

Family process, alteration in
Grieving, dysfunctional
Health maintenance, alteration in
Parenting, alteration in: actual or potential

Diagnosis Related Groups

Potentially applicable within all diagnosis related groups

	COPING, INEFFECTIVE
Nursing Diagnosis	**INDIVIDUAL**

Potential
Clinical Findings

Chronic anxiety, fear
Poor self-esteem
Inability to problem solve
Unrealistic perceptions
Inadequate support systems
Destructive behavior toward self or others
Alcohol proneness
High rate of accidents
Inability to seek assistance
Maladaptive behaviors
Inability to care for basic needs
Usual coping methods ineffective or unavailable

Expected
Outcomes

The patient will develop ways to cope effectively with the demands of life.

Interventions

- Assess stressors and precipitating causes of current situation.
- Work with patient to assess physical and emotional needs.
- Identify patient's coping skills, strengths, and weaknesses.
- Evaluate patient's individual insight into the problem(s).
- Identify resources available to the patient

  - satisfaction with relationships and family
  - how decisions are made
  - marital stability
  - communication and speech patterns
  - religious beliefs and practices
  - ability to organize after a crisis

- adaptation to organization and management of daily schedule change since diagnosis
- financial, educational, and cultural status
- basic physical resources (home, health care, crisis prevention, equipment needs, food, clothing)
- ability to understand
- degree of impairment and functional capacity
- developmental level of functioning
- alcohol, smoking, eating patterns

- Encourage patient to mobilize available external and internal resources (specify available ones).
- Work with patient to identify unmet needs; explore alternatives to meet them.
- Provide a quiet environment.
- Evaluate effects of prescribed medications.
- Listen therapeutically (e.g., use open-ended sentences, restatements, validation of information).
- Provide emotional support/honest reassurance to individual and family (e.g., answer all questions honestly without statements of false assurance).
- Be consistent in all approaches to the patient.
- Do not encourage or reinforce any maladaptive behavior patient may be exhibiting (e.g., blaming others, aggression, withdrawal).
- Teach use of "I" statements to state feelings and needs.
- Provide opportunity for patient to verbalize feelings and needs assertively.

- Evaluate patient's decision-making ability.
- Provide opportunity for patient to explore alternatives in decision making; teach to explore consequences of each alternative.
- Help patient begin to implement alternative actions.
- Identify negative patient behaviors; help patient to recognize and redirect negative behavior (e.g., use alternative behaviors).
- Assist patient to set and accomplish achievable goals.
- Support therapeutic contributions from appropriate professionals on the health care team (specify members consulted).
- Teach patient about medications and the importance of maintaining prescribed regimen.
- Identify patient's perception and understanding of the current situation.
- Observe for destructive behavior toward self or others; protect patient and others.
- Explain procedures, treatments in advance using simple, concise language; keep patient oriented to the here and now.
- Encourage expression of anxiety and fear; let patient know feelings of depression, anger, and confusion are normal and expected when one is ill.
- Assist patient in evaluating current life-style and stressors that can be modified to enhance better coping.

Outcome Criteria The patient copes effectively with the current situation as evidenced by active participation in decisions regarding care, expression of feelings and opinions, and verbalization of confidence to cope with the current situation (specify the situation).

Potentially Related Nursing Diagnoses

Health maintenance, alteration in
Powerlessness
Self-concept, disturbance in
Social isolation
Spiritual distress

Diagnosis Related Groups

Potentially applicable within all diagnosis related groups

DIVERSIONAL ACTIVITY, DEFICIT

Nursing Diagnosis

Potential Clinical Findings

Restlessness
Demanding behavior
Anxiety
Low self-esteem
Depression
Pain
Apathy
Nausea
Traumatic life-style change
Self-centered focus

Expected Outcomes

The patient will actively participate in planning and utilizing diversional activities (specify activities).

Interventions

- Assess physical and emotional status.
- Identify patient's areas of interest.
- Identify availability of resources (e.g., family, financial, community, cultural traditions, education, religious background).
- Avoid sensory overload by providing activities in small increments as patient can manage.
- Establish a trust relationship with patient; encourage expression of feelings.
- Listen therapeutically (e.g., encourage use of "I" statements to express feelings and needs).
- Explore the patient's perceptions of own behavior and that of others.
- Offer diversional activities such as television, reading, arts and crafts, hobbies, writing, physical activities, grooming.

- Encourage interest in and contact with others; allow visitors as patient's condition warrants; encourage patient to interact with staff.
- Assist patient with postdischarge diversional planning; explore senior service centers, transportation options, clubs and group activities, and contacting friends.

Outcome Criteria

The patient has adequate diversional activity as evidenced by participation in activities (specify activities), verbalization of satisfaction with diversional involvement, and concrete plans for future activities and involvement with outside interests.

Potentially Related Nursing Diagnoses

All diagnoses

Diagnosis Related Groups

Potentially applicable within all diagnosis related groups

FAMILY PROCESS, ALTERATION IN

Nursing Diagnosis

Potential Clinical Findings

Optimally functioning family in crisis not seeking help appropriately

Not meeting physical, emotional, spiritual needs of family

Inability to adapt to change

Inability to express or accept wide range of feelings

Inadequate crisis management

Ineffective communication patterns

Interruption of normal family routine

Delayed completion of family developmental tasks

Anger

Guilt

Ineffective family decision making

Expected Outcomes

The family will exhibit appropriate functional behaviors in present crisis.

Interventions

- Evaluate the current situation (crisis or chronic, physical or emotional).
- Identify developmental stage of family unit.
- Identify family resources

  - satisfaction with relationships
  - how decisions are made and by whom
  - hierarchy (who sets limits/discipline, who helps with what tasks)
  - marital stability
  - communication patterns
  - relationship with extended family
  - religious beliefs and practices
  - ability to organize after a crisis

- adaptation to organization and management of daily schedule changes since diagnosis
- sacrifices necessary for family function and feelings regarding sacrifices
- expectations of each member and family roles
- financial, educational, and cultural status
- basic physical resources (home, health care, crisis prevention, equipment needs, clothing and food)

- Utilize internal and external family resources as available and as appropriate.
- Establish a trusting relationship with the family and maintain consistency in all interactions with the family.
- Reduce environmental stress (e.g., provide a quiet atmosphere, make few interruptions).
- Provide reliable information; correct misconceptions.
- Teach effective communication patterns.
- Provide opportunity for family to practice new communication patterns (e.g., role playing, family meetings).
- Encourage use of "I" statements to express feelings and needs.
- Encourage family members to accept feelings of others as valid.
- Identify to family the consequences of inappropriate, inconsistent behavior.
- Teach problem-solving techniques.

- Provide opportunity for family to participate in problem solving (e.g., planning alternatives).
- Identify the precipitating event (e.g., illness, trauma) that has caused the crisis; determine the impact of the change on the family.
- Allow ventilation of feelings of helplessness, anger, sorrow, and confusion; give empathy and support without judgment.
- Articulate the problem as you understand it and validate it with all family members.
- Lend perspective and give feedback to assist family in viewing the problem from each other's point of view.
- Review all alternatives available and outside resources as indicated.

Outcome Criteria

The family exhibits appropriate functional behaviors as evidenced by effective communication within family unit, effective use of problem-solving techniques, progress in developmental tasks, utilization of internal and external resources (specify available resources), and verbalization of satisfaction with adaptation to the current situation.

Potentially Related Nursing Diagnoses

Coping, ineffective family: compromised

Grieving, anticipatory/dysfunctional

Knowledge deficit (specify)

Parenting, alteration in: actual or potential

Diagnosis Related Groups

Potentially applicable within all diagnosis related groups

Nursing Diagnosis **FEAR**

Potential Clinical Findings

Apprehensive
Scared
Jittery
Demanding behavior, aggressive
Feelings of loss of control
Headache, nausea and vomiting
Elevated blood pressure
Tachycardia
Tachypnea
Diaphoresis
Increased muscle tension
Rigid posture
Feelings of panic
Increased verbalization
Increased questioning
Lack of eye contact

Expected Outcomes

The patient will identify the source of the fear and participate in steps to reduce or alleviate it.

Interventions

● Identify and assess with the patient

- intensity of fear
- nature of fear
- precipitating factors
- aggravating factors
- alleviating factors

● Reduce/eliminate outside stimuli.
● Listen to the patient; accept the validity of patient's fear-producing perceptions.
● Provide honest reassurance.
● Provide reliable information (i.e., explain tasks and procedures accurately at the patient's level of understanding).
● Help resolve acute fear crisis

- do not leave patient alone
- be aware and in control of personal emotions and actions (do not project staff fears and attitudes to the patient)
- use specific interventions to establish immediate and firm control (e.g., encourage slow, deep breathing; distraction techniques)
- give commands in simple, direct language; repeat all comments as necessary
- focus patient attention on rational perceptions
- promote patient control of the situation when possible; allow patient to plan and participate in care

● Provide diversional activities; focus on the use of alleviating factors.

Outcome Criteria

The patient identifies the source of the fear and alleviates the threat as evidenced by increased comfort, relaxed affect, and plans to avoid precipitating and aggravating factors.

Potentially Related Nursing Diagnoses

All diagnoses

Diagnosis Related Groups

Potentially applicable within all diagnosis related groups

FLUID VOLUME, ALTERATION IN: EXCESS

Nursing Diagnosis

Potential Clinical Findings

Rales
Edema
Ventricular gallop
Increased central venous pressure
Shortness of breath
Increased abdominal girth
Anxiety
Lethargy
Moist breath sounds
Restlessness
Disorientation
Venous engorgement
Poor skin turgor
Coughing
Cyanosis
Pallor
Dysuria
Oliguria
Intake greater than output
Weight gain

Expected Outcomes

The patient will regain optimal fluid balance.

Interventions

- Do a complete history and physical assessment (including intake and output during the past 24 hours).
- Place in position of comfort; raise head of bed as tolerated, supporting patient's arms to decrease shoulder muscle fatigue; change position every 2 hours as necessary.
- Evaluate effects of prescribed oxygen and medications.
- Provide a cool, dry environment.
- Monitor

  − intake and output

- daily weight
- edema (record and report increases)
- level of consciousness
- vital signs (include characteristics of respirations: depth, rate, use of accessory muscles, etc.)
- bowel movements
- skin integrity
- x-ray reports
- abdominal girth
- lab results; report significant values

  * ABGs
  * chem profile
  * CBC
  * diff
  * sed rate
  * electrolytes
  * digoxin level (if indicated)
  * urine (for UA, osmolarity, and electrolytes)
  * BUN
  * creatinine

- Anticipate needs; avoid patient anxiety.
- Provide for uninterrupted rest periods.
- Restrict fluids as ordered.
- Provide low-sodium diet as ordered; offer small portions to decrease cardiac workload.
- Promote activity as tolerated.
- Prevent constipation (e.g., provide bulk in diet; evaluate effectiveness of stool softeners, laxatives).

Outcome Criteria The patient has regained optimal fluid balance as evidenced by elastic skin, no edema, clear breath sounds, lab values within normal limits, and balanced intake/output record.

Potentially Related Nursing Diagnoses

Activity intolerance, actual or potential
Breathing pattern, ineffective
Cardiac output, alteration in: decreased
Mobility, impaired physical
Tissue perfusion, alteration in
Urinary elimination, alteration in patterns

Diagnosis Related Groups

- Diseases and Disorders of the Nervous System (e.g., craniotomy, traumatic stupor and coma)
- Diseases and Disorders of the Circulatory System (e.g., heart failure, cardiothoracic procedures)
- Diseases and Disorders of the Respiratory System (e.g., pleural effusion, pulmonary edema)
- Diseases and Disorders of the Digestive System (e.g., digestive malignancy, GI obstruction)
- Diseases and Disorders of the Hepatobiliary System and Pancreas (e.g., cirrhosis and alcoholic hepatitis; major pancreas, liver, and shunt procedures)
- Diseases and Disorders of the Musculoskeletal System and Connective Tissues (e.g., connective tissue disorders, septic arthritis)
- Endocrine, Nutritional, and Metabolic Diseases and Disorders (e.g., adrenal and pituitary procedures, thyroid procedures)
- Diseases and Disorders of the Kidney and Urinary Tract (e.g., renal failure, urethral stricture)

FLUID VOLUME DEFICIT, ACTUAL OR POTENTIAL

Nursing Diagnosis

Potential Clinical Findings

Poor skin turgor
Sallow appearance
Dry mucous membranes
Output greater than intake
Weight loss
Nausea and vomiting
Weakness
Fatigue
Dizziness
Tremors
Concentrated urine
Dysuria
Oliguria
Orthostatic hypotension
Polyuria

Expected Outcomes

Potential: The patient will *maintain* optimal fluid volume balance.

Actual: The patient will *regain* optimal fluid balance.

Interventions

- Do complete history and physical assessment (including intake and output for the past 24 hours).
- Assess for insensible fluid loss (i.e., diaphoresis)
- Monitor

  - intake and output
  - specific gravity
  - daily weight
  - orthostatic vital signs
  - temperature
  - level of consciousness and behavior
  - diet

- skin turgor, oral mucosa
- lung sounds and respirations
- Observe lab results and report significant values (be alert to the fact that dehydration will cause hemoconcentration and will increase some lab values)
  - UA
  - urine osmolarity and electrolytes
  - CBC
  - serum electrolytes
  - chem profile
  - BUN
  - creatinine
- Administer IV fluids and replace nasogastric loss as ordered.
- Evaluate effects of prescribed medications.
- Promote fluid intake unless contraindicated.
- Maintain effective skin care regimen.
- Assist patient with out-of-bed activity.
- Teach patient signs and symptoms of dehydration (specifically related to the patient's medical diagnosis).
- Teach patient about prescribed medications and the importance of maintaining regimen.

Outcome Criteria

Potential: The patient maintains fluid volume balance as evidenced by warm, elastic skin; moist oral mucosa; and balanced intake/output record.

Actual:	The patient regains optimal fluid balance as evidenced by lab values within normal limits; warm, elastic skin; moist oral mucosa; and balanced intake/output record.

Potentially Related Nursing Diagnoses

Bowel elimination, alteration in: diarrhea/constipation

Nutrition, alteration in: less than body requirements

Skin integrity, impairment of: potential

Tissue perfusion, alteration in

Urinary elimination, alteration in patterns

Diagnosis Related Groups

- Diseases and Disorders of the Respiratory System (e.g., respiratory infections and inflammations, COPD)
- Diseases and Disorders of the Circulatory System (e.g., OR procedure on circulatory system, shock)
- Diseases and Disorders of the Digestive System (e.g., hemorrhage, inflammatory bowel disease)
- Diseases and Disorders of the Kidney and Urinary Tract (e.g., kidney and urinary tract infections, urinary stones)
- Burns

| Nursing Diagnosis | **GAS EXCHANGE, IMPAIRED** |

**Potential
Clinical Findings**

Air hunger
Restlessness
Fear
Cyanosis
Tachypnea
Confusion
Tachycardia
Dysrhythmias
Anxiety
Retractions
Using accessory respiratory muscles
Nausea
Dizziness
Numbness and tingling of extremities

**Expected
Outcomes**

The patient will exhibit adequate gas exchange.

Interventions

- Maintain a patent airway.
- Place in position of comfort.
- Maintain a cool, moist air flow in the room.
- Do a physical assessment.
- Monitor

  - vital signs
  - respiratory rate, depth, and rhythm
  - intake and output
  - daily weight
  - changes in behavior and level of consciousness
  - x-ray reports
  - lab results; report significant values

    * ABGs
    * chem profile
    * CBC
    * sed rate

* electrolytes
* urinalysis
* sputum C&S, gram stain, and AFB
* theophylline level if indicated
- Evaluate effects of prescribed medications, oxygen, respiratory treatments, and IV therapy.
- Schedule and pace patient's activities to minimize oxygen requirements; allow adequate rest periods.
- Teach pursed-lip breathing and proper disposal of secretions.
- Provide oral hygiene.
- Teach patient about prescribed medications and the importance of maintaining regimen.

Outcome Criteria

The patient exhibits adequate gas exchange as evidenced by lab values indicating acid-base balance, being alert and oriented with appropriate response to commands, verbalization of increased comfort and lack of air hunger, and warm dry skin with no cyanosis.

Potentially Related Nursing Diagnoses

All diagnoses

Diagnosis Related Groups

- Diseases and Disorders of the Nervous System (e.g., craniotomy, spinal disorders and injuries)
- Diseases and Disorders of the Circulatory System (e.g., cardiac arrest, coronary bypass)
- Diseases and Disorders of the Respiratory System (e.g., pulmonary embolism, respiratory failure)

- Diseases and Disorders of the Digestive System (e.g., digestive malignancy, GI hemorrhage)
- Endocrine, Nutritional, and Metabolic Diseases and Disorders (e.g., diabetes, nutritional and miscellaneous metabolic disorders)
- Diseases and Disorders of the Musculoskeletal System and Connective Tissues (e.g., bone diseases and septic arthropathies, fractures of femur)
- Infectious and Parasitic Diseases (e.g., septicemia, viral illnesses, and fever of unknown origin)
- Myeloproliferative Diseases and Disorders, Poorly Differentiated Malignancy and other Neoplasms (e.g., lymphoma or leukemia, chemotherapy)
- Injury, Poisoning, and Toxic Effects of Drugs (e.g., allergic reactions, toxic effects of drugs)
- Substance Use and Induced, Organic Mental Disorders (e.g., drug dependence, alcohol- and substance-induced organic mental syndrome)

Nursing Diagnosis **GRIEVING, ANTICIPATORY**

**Potential
Clinical Findings**
Changes in libido
Sadness
Sorrow
Crying
Altered sleep patterns
Anger
Inappropriate behavior
Appetite fluctuations
Weight changes
Verbalizing anticipated loss

**Expected
Outcomes**
The patient will verbalize feelings about anticipated loss and will move through the grieving process.

Interventions
- Identify individual and family perceptions of the anticipated loss (stage of grieving).
- Encourage and promote verbalization of feelings; acknowledge and accept the feelings as valid.
- Evaluate internal and external resources available to the patient

    – satisfaction with relationships
    – how decisions are made and by whom
    – expectations of self and others
    – marital stability
    – communication patterns
    – relationship with extended and immediate family
    – religious beliefs and practices
    – ability to organize after a crisis
    – adaptation to organization and management of daily schedule changes since diagnosis
    – financial, educational, and cultural status

- basic physical resources (home, health care, crisis prevention, equipment needs, clothing and food)
- Encourage family unit and individuals to focus on their own strengths.
- Encourage mobilization and use of internal and external resources (specify available resources).
- Provide factual information, including an explanation of the grieving process, according to patient and family readiness.
- Ensure privacy.
- Evaluate decision-making abilities.
- Provide opportunity to explore alternatives; teach patient to explore consequences of each alternative.
- Assist patient to choose alternatives and plan for the future.
- Encourage family and individuals to continue their lives without feeling guilty.
- Suggest outside interests.
- Provide information on support groups and outside agencies of mutual interest.
- Identify potential loss and meaning of loss to the person.
- Assess how patient is handling the anticipated loss, what coping behaviors are evident.
- Provide realistic feedback and lend perspective as required to correct distorted perceptions.
- Identify specific problems anticipated by the loss and assist patient in recognizing alternatives.
- Include significant others to support patient in dealing with the situation.

Outcome Criteria

The patient moves through the grieving process as evidenced by verbalization of feelings about the anticipated loss and planning for the future.

Potentially Related Nursing Diagnoses

Coping, family: potential for growth
Family process, alteration in
Knowledge deficit (specify)

Diagnosis Related Groups

Potentially applicable within all diagnosis related groups

| **Nursing Diagnosis** | **GRIEVING, DYSFUNCTIONAL** |

Potential Clinical Findings

Verbalization of loss
Denial of loss
Changes in libido
Altered sleep pattern
Appetite fluctuations
Decreased activity
Disruption of ADL
Regression
Crying
Sadness
Reliving past experiences
Apathy
Depression
Disheveled appearance

Expected Outcomes

The patient will exhibit adaptive grieving behaviors.

Interventions

- Determine individual's perceptions of the loss.
- Assess emotional and mental status (including physical appearance and presentation).
- Provide time for patient to express feelings about the loss; accept feeling statements as valid.
- Encourage use of "I" statements to state needs and wants.
- Assess patient's internal and external resources

  - satisfaction with relationships
  - how decisions are made, and by whom
  - expectations of self and others
  - marital stability
  - communication patterns
  - relationships with extended and immediate family

- religious beliefs and practices
- ability to organize after a crisis
- adaptation to organization and management of daily schedule changes since diagnosis
- financial, educational, and cultural status
- basic physical resources (home, health care, crisis prevention, equipment needs, clothing and food)

- Identify patient's stage of grieving.
- Encourage mobilization and use of available internal and external resources.
- Provide diversional activities; help broaden patient's focus.
- Identify with patient consequences of maladaptive behavior; explore alternatives of appropriate behavior.
- Provide opportunity for patient to test alternative behaviors.
- Assist patient to continue to utilize support systems during the entire grieving process.
- Encourage family and individuals to continue their lives without feeling guilty.
- Refer patient/family to appropriate members of the health care team for follow-up.
- Explore previous unresolved losses and how patient dealt with them.
- Educate about normalcy of feelings and process of grief.
- Permit expression of anger and set limits for destructive behavior.
- Identify cultural factors that may inhibit grieving.

Outcome Criteria The patient exhibits adaptive grieving behaviors such as appropriate expression of feelings, participation in ADL, affect appropriate to surrounding conditions, and active participation in planning for the future.

Potentially Related Nursing Diagnoses Family process, alteration in
Knowledge deficit (specify)
Social isolation

Diagnosis Related Groups Potentially applicable within all diagnosis related groups

HEALTH MAINTENANCE, ALTERATION IN

Nursing Diagnosis

Potential Clinical Findings

Impaired cognitive thoughts and perceptions
Impaired mobility
Activity intolerance
Impaired communication
Lack of resources
Financial crisis
Lack of knowledge

Expected Outcomes

The patient will be able to meet health needs.

Interventions

- Assess the source and extent of the alteration.
- Evaluate resources

  - financial status
  - education
  - religion
  - extended family
  - living situation
  - cultural traditions
  - community

- Explore with patient and family alternatives available for health maintenance (e.g., in-home care, nursing facility, transportation).
- Provide adaptive equipment and necessary instruction for use (e.g., walker, oxygen, hospital bed).
- Provide referrals and follow-up with community agencies.
- Allow time for patient and family interaction regarding arrangements for health maintenance.
- Teach patient about prescribed medications and the importance of maintaining regimen.

Outcome Criteria The patient is meeting health needs as evidenced by successful demonstration of all health management skills (specify, e.g., ability to recognize threats to health, receiving and taking medication) and verbalization of satisfaction with health management arrangements.

Potentially Related Nursing Diagnoses All diagnoses

Diagnosis Related Groups Potentially applicable within all diagnosis related groups

HOME MAINTENANCE MANAGEMENT, IMPAIRED

Nursing Diagnosis

Potential Clinical Findings

Impaired mobility
Disorientation
Unkempt appearance
Household members express difficulty in providing patient care
Unavailable resources
Impaired sensory perception
Knowledge deficit
Financial crisis
Unkempt or unsuitable home environment

Expected Outcome

The patient will be maintained at home safely.

Interventions

- Assess the source and extent of the impairment.
- Identify resources

  - financial status
  - education
  - religion
  - extended family
  - living situation
  - cultural traditions
  - community options of assistance
  - transportation

- Assist patient and family to recognize need for assistance in the home.
- Provide information about available, appropriate resources.
- Explore with patient and family alternatives available (e.g., home care, transportation, meals brought in).
- Provide adaptive equipment and necessary instruction for use (e.g., walker, wheelchair, oxygen, suction equipment).

- Encourage verbalization of feelings regarding loss of independence.
- Provide referrals and follow-up with other members of health care team (e.g., physical therapy, respiratory therapy) and with community agencies.
- Allow time for patient and family interaction regarding arrangements for home maintenance management.
- Evaluate living situation for safety hazards and provide safe alternatives.
- Teach patient about prescribed medications and the importance of maintaining regimen.

Outcome Criteria

The patient is safely managing at home as evidenced by absence of safety hazards, verbalized satisfaction with home management, appropriate use of adaptive equipment (specify), and appropriate utilization of resources (specify, e.g., meals brought in, bathing assistance).

Potentially Related Nursing Diagnoses

All diagnoses

Diagnosis Related Groups

Potentially applicable within all diagnosis related groups

Nursing Diagnosis	# INJURY, POTENTIAL FOR
Potential Clinical Findings	Confusion Agitation Weakness Very young or very old Diminished pain sensation Impaired judgment Impaired skin integrity Sensory deprivation Immunosuppression Altered level of consciousness Destructive behavior Impaired mobility Frequent contact with potentially hazardous equipment
Expected Outcomes	The patient will be free from injury (e.g., poisoning, suffocation, trauma, infection).
Interventions	• Assess potential sources of injury. • Evaluate physical and mental status, risk of further injury, infection (related to trauma, surgical or disease processes). • Promote patient safety

- demonstrate use of call system; place within reach of patient
- anticipate needs; answer calls promptly
- use restraints if necessary
- keep siderails "up"
- assist patient with activity (both in and out of bed)
- recheck patient position frequently
- provide adequate lighting
- lock movable furniture into position

- check adequate grounding of electrical equipment
- minimize obstacles
- avoid improper use of equipment in patient areas
- provide nonskid, well-fitting footwear
- offer regular bathroom privileges (around the clock)
- remove potentially injurious items from patient areas (e.g., sharp objects, medications)

- Follow aseptic protocol when caring for wounds.
- Maintain isolation protocol for immunosuppressed patients.
- Inform visitors/family of potential risks and necessary precautions.

Outcome Criteria

The patient is free from injury as evidenced by intact physiologic integrity (e.g., lack of infection, trauma).

Potentially Related Nursing Diagnoses

Mobility, impaired physical
Sensory-perceptual alteration
Violence, potential for

Diagnosis Related Groups

- Diseases and Disorders of the Nervous System (e.g., multiple sclerosis, transient ischemic attacks)
- Diseases and Disorders of the Eye (e.g., neurologic eye disorders)
- Diseases and Disorders of the Ear, Nose, and Throat (e.g., disequilibrium)
- Diseases and Disorders of the Respiratory System (e.g., pneumothorax, major chest trauma)

- Diseases and Disorders of the Circulatory System (e.g., atherosclerosis, peripheral vascular disorders)
- Diseases and Disorders of the Digestive System (e.g., minor small and large bowel procedures, anal procedures)
- Diseases and Disorders of the Hepatobiliary System and Pancreas (e.g., biliary tract procedures, cirrhosis and alcoholic hepatitis)
- Diseases and Disorders of the Musculoskeletal System and Connective Tissues (e.g., amputations, knee procedures)
- Endocrine, Nutritional, and Metabolic Diseases and Disorders (e.g., diabetes, skin grafts and wound debridement)
- Diseases and Disorders of the Kidney and Urinary Tract (e.g., renal failure; kidney, ureter, major bladder procedure for neoplasm)
- Diseases and Disorders of the Male Reproductive System (e.g., transurethral prostatectomy, penis procedures)
- Diseases and Disorders of the Female Reproductive System (e.g., malignancy of female reproductive system, infections of female reproductive system)
- Myeloproliferative Diseases and Disorders, Poorly Differentiated Malignancy and Other Neoplasms (e.g., radiotherapy, chemotherapy)
- Infectious and Parasitic Diseases (e.g., septicemia, fever of unknown origin)

- Mental Diseases and Disorders (e.g., disorders of personality and impulse control, depressive neuroses)
- Injury, Poisoning, and Toxic Effects of Drugs (e.g., alcohol- and substance-induced organic mental syndrome, toxic effects of drugs)

KNOWLEDGE DEFICIT
Nursing Diagnosis (SPECIFY)

Potential
Clinical Findings
Inadequate knowledge base
Verbalization of inadequate knowledge
Verbalization of misinformation
Making uninformed decisions
Seeking information

Expected
Outcomes
The patient will verbalize and/or demonstrate understanding of established learning objectives (specify objectives).

Interventions
- Identify specific learning needs.
- Assess readiness and motivation to learn, including culture and language, preconceptions, educational level, and attention span.
- Begin by addressing the learner's priorities.
- Validate identified learning needs with the patient.
- Work with the learner to establish specific, measurable learning objectives.
- Plan the teaching-learning process.
- Provide an environment conducive to learning (e.g., room without distractions, adequate lighting).
- Utilize a variety of teaching methods
  - written material
  - oral presentation
  - audio-visual aids
  - repetition
  - demonstration/return demonstration (patient performs techniques/ skills taught by nurse)
- Present information in small increments.

- Be alert to and utilize teachable moments (e.g., during routine care; spontaneous informal teaching as questions arise).
- Reinforce all attempts to learn.
- Devise guidelines for evaluation (e.g., verbalization, return demonstration, compliance).

Outcome Criteria

The patient has met established learning objectives as evidenced by successful completion of return demonstration (specify objectives) and verbalization of comprehension of information presented (specify information/objectives).

Potentially Related Nursing Diagnoses

All diagnoses

Diagnosis Related Groups

Potentially applicable within all diagnosis related groups

MOBILITY, IMPAIRED PHYSICAL

Nursing Diagnosis

Potential Clinical Findings

Limited range of motion
Altered coordination
Weakness
Muscle atrophy
Disequilibrium
Restrictions imposed by medical regimen (from traction, casting, etc.)
Pain

Expected Outcomes

The patient will regain optimum mobility (specify patient's optimum).

Interventions

- Assess the source, extent, and implications of impairment.
- Evaluate current range of motion.
- Perform range-of-motion exercises (both active and passive) 4 times daily and prn.
- Provide good skin care; reposition at least every 2 hours.
- Assist with transfers and ambulation.
- Provide a call system adapted to patient's needs.
- If able to get out of bed, ambulate at least 3 times daily as patient tolerates; sit in chair at least 3 times daily as tolerated.
- Encourage independence (within reason).
- Instruct family about the extent of impairment and selected interventions.
- Teach patient about prescribed medications and the importance of maintaining regimen.

Outcome Criteria

The patient has regained optimum mobility as evidenced by optimal range of motion, ability to maneuver within physical limitations, verbalized pleasure in increased activity, and care-giver verbalization and demonstration of mobility maintenance (specify).

Potentially Related Nursing Diagnoses

- Activity intolerance, actual or potential
- Self-care deficit (specify level)

Diagnosis Related Groups

- Diseases and Disorders of the Nervous System (e.g., degenerative nervous system disorders, spinal disorders and injuries)
- Diseases and Disorders of the Eye (e.g., acute major eye infections, retinal procedures)
- Diseases and Disorders of the Ear, Nose, and Throat (e.g., disequilibrium, major head and neck procedures)
- Diseases and Disorders of the Circulatory System (e.g., peripheral vascular disorders, angina pectoris)
- Diseases and Disorders of the Respiratory System (e.g., COPD, simple pneumonia and pleurisy)
- Diseases and Disorders of the Digestive System (e.g., major small and large bowel procedures, inflammatory bowel disease)
- Diseases and Disorders of the Musculoskeletal System and Connective Tissues (e.g., amputations, major joint procedures)

Nursing Diagnosis ## NONCOMPLIANCE (SPECIFY)

Potential Clinical Findings

Exacerbation of symptoms
Verbalization of noncompliance
Frequent readmissions with same problems
Demanding behavior
Anger
Apathy

Expected Outcomes

The patient will comply with plan of care (specify plan).

Interventions

- Do history and physical evaluation.
- Assess source and degree of noncompliance.
- Assess learning needs. Avoid projecting behaviors that might provoke noncompliance (e.g., appearing rushed, uninterested, commanding).
- Reduce verbalized actual or perceived threats that might lead to noncompliance (e.g., altered body image, fear of toxic effects).
- Create and implement appropriate teaching plans.
- Explore with patient constructive options of compliant behavior.
- Present potentially threatening material (e.g., any plan requiring change in behavior) in small increments.
- Avoid vague, nonspecific statements; focus on reality, facts.

Outcome Criteria

The patient complies with the plan of care as evidenced by remittance of symptoms, resolution of the problem, and adherence to prescribed regimen.

Potentially Related Nursing Diagnoses	All diagnoses
Diagnosis Related Groups	Potentially applicable within all diagnosis related groups

NUTRITION, ALTERATION IN: LESS THAN BODY REQUIREMENTS

Nursing Diagnosis

Potential Clinical Findings

Weight loss
Decreased appetite
Decreased energy level
Alopecia
Dry, flaky skin with poor turgor
Nausea
Bleeding gums
Illness prone
Alteration in sleep pattern
Protruding bony prominences
Brittle nails
Weakness

Expected Outcomes

The patient will increase nutritional intake; will ingest a balanced diet.

Interventions

- Identify the reason for nutrient depletion
- Obtain actual height and weight; measure skin folds to calculate ideal weight.
- Assess

  - oral mucous membranes
  - skin color, temperature, integrity, and turgor
  - dentures for proper fit and placement for eating
  - food likes and dislikes

- Monitor

  - diagnostic procedure reports
  - lab results; report significant values

    * CBC
    * sed rate
    * chem profile

          * electrolytes
          * thyroid studies
          * UA
          * calorie counts and daily weight

       – frequency and characteristics of urine and stool

- Set an ideal weight goal agreeable to the patient.
- Evaluate effects of prescribed medications (medications may cause nutritional depletion).
- Medicate for discomfort related to feedings (e.g., nausea, pain, tremors); evaluate effects.
- Promote oral hygiene and dental care.
- Provide rest periods before meals to increase energy for eating.
- Assess effect of prescribed premeal stimulants (e.g., wine, medications, oral stimulation).
- Make mealtimes pleasant

       – provide desirable food items; alter food consistency to facilitate eating
       – allow patient participation in menu selection
       – ensure uninterrupted feeding times
       – prepare attractive meal trays
       – place patient in a comfortable position for eating
       – provide socialization

- Feed patient as necessary.
- Offer frequent, small meals.
- Provide supplemental nutrition (e.g., tube feedings, total parenteral nutrition) as needed.

Outcome Criteria

The patient has increased nutritional intake as evidenced by measurable (weekly) weight gain, normal lab values, and participation in menu planning (indicates ability to balance diet for adequate nutrient intake).

Potentially Related Nursing Diagnoses

Knowledge deficit (specify)
Self-concept, disturbance in

Diagnosis Related Groups

- Diseases and Disorders of the Nervous System (e.g., nonspecific cerebrovascular disorders, cranial and peripheral nerve disorders)
- Diseases and Disorders of the Circulatory System (e.g., atherosclerosis, cardiac congenital and valvular disorders)
- Diseases and Disorders of the Respiratory System (e.g., interstitial lung disease, respiratory neoplasms)
- Diseases and Disorders of the Digestive System (e.g., inflammatory bowel disease; esophagitis, gastroenteritis and miscellaneous digestive disorders)
- Diseases and Disorders of the Hepatobiliary System and Pancreas (e.g., major pancreas, liver, and shunt procedures; malignancies of the pancreas)
- Diseases and Disorders of the Ear, Nose, and Throat (e.g., cleft lip and palate repair; ear, nose, and throat malignancy)
- Substance Use and Induced, Organic Mental Disorders (e.g., drug dependence, alcohol dependence)
- Burns
- Mental Diseases and Disorders (e.g., depressive neuroses, disorders of personality and impulse control)

- Infectious and Parasitic Diseases (e.g., fever of unknown origin, postoperative infections)
- Myeloproliferative Diseases and Disorders, Poorly Differentiated Malignancy and Other Neoplasms (e.g., lymphoma or leukemia, chemotherapy)
- Endocrine, Nutritional, and Metabolic Diseases and Disorders (e.g., diabetes, OR procedures for obesity)
- Pregnancy, Childbirth, and the Puerperium (e.g., ectopic pregnancy, threatened abortion)
- Newborns and other Neonates with Conditions Originating in the Perinatal Period (e.g., extreme immaturity, full-term neonates with major problems)
- Diseases and Disorders of Blood and Blood Forming Organs and Immunity Disorders (e.g., reticuloendothelial and immunity disorders, splenectomy)

NUTRITION, ALTERATION IN: MORE THAN BODY REQUIREMENTS

Nursing Diagnosis

Potential Clinical Findings

Obesity
Depression
Anger
Compulsive behavior
Diaphoresis
Discomfort
Withdrawal
Overeating
Dyspnea with exertion

Expected Outcomes

The patient will decrease nutrient intake and increase activity.

Interventions

- Obtain actual height and weight; measure skin folds to calculate ideal weight.
- Identify source of food excess; review diet history

  - recent intake
  - food eaten, where and when
  - activity before and after eating
  - feelings and mood before and after eating
  - onset of obesity
  - family history of overweight

- Monitor

  - weight weekly or biweekly
  - calorie count
  - potential health problems (e.g., diabetes, hypertension)
  - lab results; report significant values

    * chem profile
    * CBC

* thyroid studies
* UA

- Provide diet counseling as patient is ready to accept it; include diet therapy, identification of behavior that leads to overeating, behavior modification, group therapy, and physical exercise.
- Facilitate compliance with prescribed diet by providing positive reinforcement.
- Promote increased physical activity as indicated.
- Provide emotional support for family and patient as they learn new behaviors.
- Encourage verbalization of feelings related to being overweight and having to learn new behaviors.
- Provide information on potential health problems (e.g., hypertension).
- Reinforce positive weight-reducing behaviors.
- Provide information on support groups and outside agencies of mutual interest.
- Refer patient to other members of the health care team as indicated (e.g., occupational therapist, nutritionist, psychiatric nurse).
- Teach patient about prescribed medications and the importance of maintaining regimen.

Outcome Criteria The patient decreases amount of food intake and increases activity as evidenced by a decrease in body weight, active participation in a regular exercise program, and verbalized satisfaction of modified behavior and weight loss.

Potentially Related Nursing Diagnoses

Coping, ineffective individual
Knowledge deficit (specify)
Self-concept, disturbance in

Diagnosis Related Groups

- Endocrine, Nutritional, and Metabolic Diseases and Disorders (e.g., thyroid procedures, nutritional and miscellaneous metabolic disorders)
- Mental Diseases and Disorders (e.g., disorders of personality and impulse control, organic disturbances and mental retardation)

NUTRITION, ALTERATION IN: POTENTIAL FOR MORE THAN BODY REQUIREMENTS

Nursing Diagnosis

Potential Clinical Findings

Recent life-style change
Social isolation
Impaired mobility
Anger
Previous history of obesity
Undisciplined eating habits
Recently diagnosed illness
Depression

Expected Outcomes

The patient will identify the potential for and interventions to prevent excess food intake.

Interventions

- Obtain patient's actual height and weight; measure skin folds to calculate ideal weight.
- Review diet history

  - recent intake
  - food eaten, where and when activity before and after eating
  - feelings before and after eating

- Monitor

  - weight
  - caloric intake
  - intake and output
  - activity
  - potential health problems (e.g., diabetes, hypertension)
  - lab results; report significant values

    * CBC
    * chem profile
    * thyroid studies
    * UA

- Provide dietary consultation as necessary.
- Teach menu planning.
- Provide emotional support for the family and patient learning new behaviors (specify behaviors, e.g., altered cooking methods, exercise, changed eating habits).
- Teach patient and family about potential problems resulting in or from nutritional excess (e.g., disease process, medication side effects, impaired mobility).
- Work with patient to develop a regimen to increase activity and decrease calorie consumption (provide opportunity for physical activity, limit snacks).
- Reinforce positive weight-control behaviors.

Outcome Criteria

The patient verbalizes the potential for an excess food intake; prevents weight gain as evidenced by maintenance of current body weight, active planning to avoid excess food intake, and participation in regular physical exercise.

Potentially Related Nursing Diagnoses

Coping, ineffective individual
Diversional activity, deficit
Knowledge deficit (specify)

Diagnosis Related Groups

- Diseases and Disorders of the Circulatory System (e.g., deep vein thrombophlebitis, peripheral vascular disorders)
- Diseases and Disorders of the Digestive System (e.g., inflammatory bowel disease, uncomplicated peptic ulcer)

- Diseases and Disorders of the Hepatobiliary System and Pancreas (e.g., total cholecystectomy, disorders of the biliary tract)
- Endocrine, Nutritional, and Metabolic Diseases and Disorders (e.g., adrenal and pituitary procedures, nutritional and miscellaneous metabolic disorders)
- Diseases and Disorders of the Kidney and Urinary Tract (e.g., renal failure, kidney transplant)
- Pregnancy, Childbirth, and the Puerperium (e.g., postpartum diagnoses without OR procedure, cesarean section)
- Mental Diseases and Disorders (e.g., neuroses except depressive, acute adjustment reaction and disturbances of psychosocial dysfunction)

ORAL MUCOUS MEMBRANE, ALTERATION IN

Nursing Diagnosis

Potential Clinical Findings

Dry mucous membranes
Poor skin turgor
Pain
Poorly fitting dentures
Recent oral surgery
Tobacco, alcohol/drug abuse
Recent chemotherapy
Coma
Agitation
Presence of endotracheal tube
Young or old age
Bleeding gums
Oral lesions

Expected Outcomes

The patient will regain moist, intact mucous membrane.

Interventions

- Assess

  - oral membrane (color, moisture, masses, ulcerations, odor)
  - teeth (number and condition)
  - protruded tongue (deviations from midline and uvula symmetry)
  - voice (hoarseness)
  - gums (color, moisture, ulcerations, recession)

- Identify tobacco, drug/alcohol abuse.
- Provide appropriate mouth care; record exact amounts of ingredients used and care schedule.
- Evaluate effects of prescribed medications.
- Monitor lab results and report significant values

  - CBC
  - sed rate

- chem profile
- vitamin levels
- Provide adequate nutrition in attractive portions that can be consumed without causing further oral irritation.
- Develop a communication system if patient is unable to speak.
- Give valid reassurance; alleviate patient anxiety.
- Remove irritating dentures between meals.
- Teach patient to do good oral hygiene.
- Instruct the patient in the benefits of avoiding tobacco and alcohol.
- Teach patient about prescribed medications and importance of maintaining regimen.

Outcome Criteria

- The patient has pink, moist, intact oral mucous membrane.
- The patient eats and drinks with minimum discomfort.

Potentially Related Nursing Diagnoses

- Comfort, alteration in: pain
- Fluid volume deficit, actual or potential
- Nutrition, alteration in: less than body requirements

Diagnosis Related Groups

Potentially applicable within all diagnosis related groups

PARENTING, ALTERATION IN: ACTUAL OR POTENTIAL

Nursing Diagnosis

Potential Clinical Findings

Parent

- unrealistic expectations
- lack of bonding behavior
- inappropriate stimulation
- unresponsive to child's needs
- history of abuse as a child
- inadequate support systems
- physical or mental illness
- stress
- social isolation
- teenage parents
- knowledge deficit
- skill deficit
- inadequate role models
- incomplete bonding process
- sadness

Child

- abuse
- abandonment
- failure to thrive
- delayed growth and development
- frequent illnesses

Expected Outcomes

- The parents will express feelings regarding presence and care of their child.
- The parents will identify actual or potential risk factors that may interfere with parenting skills.
- The parents will demonstrate positive bonding behavior (e.g., playing with child; gently touching, stroking child).

Interventions
- Observe parents' behavior
  - responses to child's crying, laughing, etc.
  - feeding child
  - interactions
- Evaluate growth and development stages of parents and child.
- Assess child for indications of possible abuse (physical, emotional, sexual); report suspicions to the proper authority; attend to medical needs.
- Assess parental concern and involvement of other family members in childrearing.
- Assess parents' internal and external resources
  - satisfaction with relationships
  - how decisions are made and by whom
  - hierarchy (who sets limits/discipline, who helps with what tasks)
  - marital stability
  - communication patterns
  - relationships with extended family
  - religious beliefs and practices
  - ability to organize after a crisis
  - adaptation to organization and management of daily schedule changes
  - sacrifices necessary for family function; feelings regarding sacrifices; expectations of each member
  - financial, educational, and cultural status
  - basic physical resources (home, health care, crisis prevention, equipment needs, clothing and food)

- Mobilize and utilize available resources to help family cope with current situation.
- Provide emotional support for parents (e.g., listen therapeutically, accept their feelings as valid, assure they are not alone).
- Provide appropriate information; correct misconceptions (e.g., child growth and development, parenting skills).
- Teach parents the importance of bonding behaviors and how to exhibit them (e.g., touching child, calling child by name, eye contact); provide opportunity for parents to practice and utilize them (e.g., role playing, return demonstration, time with child).
- Teach parents appropriate care-giving behaviors in response to child's needs (e.g., feeding, rest/activity, toilet training), and provide opportunity for them to practice them (e.g., involve in child's care, plan for child's needs).
- Identify with parents risk factors that may interfere with parenting skills.
- Explore with parents alternative adaptive behaviors that will decrease interference from identified risk factors; identify consequences of each alternative.
- Point out to parents inappropriate parenting behaviors; explore alternatives; teach consequences of each one.

- Teach parents it is all right for them to experience all emotions, but they must respond to them with appropriate behavior (i.e., feelings are not wrong but some behavior can be wrong).
- Teach effective communication skills and provide opportunity to practice them (e.g., in role playing, parent-child interaction).
- Encourage parents to use "I" statements to state wants and needs, and to accept feeling statements of others as valid.
- Reinforce positive changes in behavior.
- Consult with family therapist and other health professionals as indicated; stress adequate follow-up visits.
- Provide information on support groups and outside agencies of mutual interest.

Outcome Criteria

- The parents verbalize feelings and needs.
- The parents demonstrate positive parenting behaviors (e.g., talking/singing to child, rocking/playing with child).
- The parents can identify at least one high risk factor that interferes with child care, and have a plan to reduce the risk.

Potentially Related Nursing Diagnoses

Coping, ineffective individual/family
Family process, alteration in
Knowledge deficit (specify)

Diagnosis Related Groups

- Pregnancy, Childbirth, and the Puerperium (e.g., cesarean section with complications; antepartum diagnoses with medical complications)
- Mental Diseases and Disorders (e.g., depressive neuroses; psychoses)
- Newborns and other Neonates with Conditions Originating in the Perinatal Period (e.g., full-term neonate with major problems, normal newborns)

POWERLESSNESS

Verbalization of having no control over situation

Believes events are subject to fate, chance, luck rather than one's choices

Perceives others as more powerful and in control of events

External rather than internal locus of control orientation

Believes in inability to help self

Believes personal behavior cannot affect outcome

Passivity, hesitancy, indecisiveness

Inability to seek information about treatment or self-care

Reluctance to express feelings

Apathy

Low self-esteem, feeling of worthlessness

Helplessness

**Expected
Outcomes** The patient will demonstrate the ability to identify and make choices concerning own health care.

Interventions
- Identify beliefs of individual concerning control issues

  - ability to effect outcome by choice, behavior
  - others seen as more powerful (more in control)
  - amount of choice individual feels s/he has

- Determine patient's usual coping to enable patient's participation in decision making and care.
- Eliminate unpredictability of events by informing patient of schedule,

treatments, expected disease process, people who will be coming, etc.
- Give anticipatory guidance to help patient prepare for events.
- Explore how the problem and treatment will affect patient's life.
- Determine patient's perception of the value of changing own beliefs, behavior, etc.
- Explore the influence significant other(s) and family have on patient.
- Assist patient in setting realistic goals and defining the steps to be taken to achieve expected outcome.
- Identify factors contributing to the present state of helplessness and suggest alternatives.
- Encourage patient's verbalization of feelings of helplessness, hopelessness, frustration, and anxiety.
- Reiterate to patient, "You do have some control. These are some of your choices. Let's talk about the probable outcome of each."
- Modify the environment to increase patient control (e.g., put call light in reach; decrease waiting time for treatments, meals, etc.; inform patient of time schedule).
- Have patient write a list of specific questions for the physician prior to MD's visit.
- Keep patient informed of progress during treatments; find out if there are any questions.
- Give patient as much responsibility as can be handled; evaluate on an ongoing basis for need to change degree of responsibility.
- Observe for verbal and nonverbal clues that patient is ready to learn

more about own care; initiate patient teaching in organized, sequential manner.
- Provide patient with as much information as possible about own illness, treatment, goals, changes, etc.
- Reinforce positive behavior demonstrating taking control of the situation, making choices, planning ahead, etc.
- Identify with patient negative perceptions and behaviors and how they decrease feelings of power.
- Reduce environmental stress (e.g., noise, interruptions).
- Mobilize and utilize support systems (specify available resources).
- Provide positive activities suited to the patient's abilities and limitations.
- Encourage decision making; begin with noncritical situations that allow a change of mind if necessary.

Outcome Criteria

The patient experiences an increase in personal power as evidenced by expression of needs and wants, active decision making, and carrying out ADL.

Potentially Related Nursing Diagnoses

Coping, ineffective individual
Fear
Knowledge deficit (specify)
Self-concept, disturbance in
Spiritual distress

Diagnosis Related Groups

Potentially applicable within all diagnosis related groups

Nursing Diagnosis	**RAPE-TRAUMA SYNDROME**

Potential Clinical Findings

Verbalization of rape
Anxiety
Guilt
Shame
Fear
Distrust
Anger
Feelings of violation
Ecchymosis
Edema
Lacerations
Contusions

Expected Outcomes

The patient will verbalize feelings and will be aware of available support systems.

Interventions

- Provide a private room and stay with the patient. Prior to examination, advise the patient not to

  - bathe or shower
  - brush teeth
  - comb hair
  - wash clothing

- Explain importance of physical material as evidence for possible prosecution.
- Explain all procedures beforehand and assist with physician's examination; pay particular attention to

  - general physical condition (bruises, lacerations, condition of clothing)
  - patient's statements of the incident
  - taking fingernail scrapings, retrieving loose hair or clothing fi-

bers for further testing as necessary
- obtaining smears (vaginal, cervical, anal, oral) for analysis (motile sperm, cultures, etc.)

- Do an emotional assessment; note major concerns (e.g., spouse, family, friends, effect of the attack on personal relationships).
- Arrange for relatives or friends to be with patient if desired.
- Discuss the situation with patient's friends and/or family *(with patient's permission)*; emphasize patient's feelings about the experience and fear of how significant others will respond to news of the attack.
- Reinforce to patient and family/ friend(s) that responsibility for attack lies with the attacker, not with patient.
- Encourage patient to verbalize feelings; listen therapeutically and allow adequate time for patient to talk about the trauma.
- Arrange for rape crisis counseling. Encourage patient to follow through on appointments.
- Provide information regarding possibilities of pregnancy and/or venereal disease; focus teaching on symptoms and alternatives of treatment.
- Arrange for patient to leave with someone with whom s/he will feel safe.

Outcome Criteria

The patient expresses feelings, interacts with family/friends; expresses willingness to follow through on appointments with a crisis counselor.

Potentially Related Nursing Diagnoses

Fear
Grieving, anticipatory
Powerlessness
Self-concept, disturbance in
Sexual dysfunction

Diagnosis Related Groups

- Diseases and Disorders of the Digestive System (e.g., anal procedures, miscellaneous digestive disorders)
- Diseases and Disorders of the Kidney and Urinary Tract (e.g., minor bladder procedures, kidney and urinary tract signs and symptoms)
- Diseases and Disorders of the Male Reproductive System (e.g., inflammation of the male reproductive system, penis procedures)
- Diseases and Disorders of the Female Reproductive System (e.g., infections of the female reproductive system; vagina, cervix, and vulva procedures)
- Mental Diseases and Disorders (e.g., acute adjustment reaction and disturbances of psychosocial dysfunction; neuroses except depressive)

SELF-CARE DEFICIT (SPECIFY LEVEL)

Nursing Diagnosis

Potential Clinical Findings

Depression
Anxiety
Fear
Confusion
Impaired mobility
Muscle atrophy
Weakness
Paralysis
Compromised respiratory status
Compromised circulatory status
Inability to complete ADL

Expected Outcomes

The patient will be able to adapt and complete self-care tasks (specify level).

Interventions

- Evaluate

  - the source, extent, and implications of the deficit
  - patient's understanding of the deficit
  - patient's coping and adaptation abilities

- Provide physical care until patient is able to manage unaided.
- Keep self-care and personal items within reach of the patient.
- Teach alternative methods of performing tasks as feasible (e.g., shower instead of tub bath; nonchildproof lids of prescriptions; sitting down to dress).
- Teach patient to use adaptive devices as needed.
- Involve family and/or care givers in teaching and patient care.

- Assist patient and family in realistic goal-setting and planning self-care at home.
- Work with patient to establish care routine, allowing adequate rest periods between tasks.
- Encourage patient to verbalize feelings related to deficits in self-care; accept patient's feelings as valid.
- Provide emotional support for patient and family learning new methods of task completion.
- Praise all efforts and accomplishments in self-care.
- Consult with physical/occupational therapists and other members of the health care team as appropriate.
- Work to ensure adequate follow-up and care in the community and at home.

Outcome Criteria

The patient has adapted and completes self-care tasks as evidenced by carrying out own ADL with some assistance as necessary; verbalizes satisfaction with physical abilities.

Potentially Related Nursing Diagnoses

Health maintenance, alteration in
Home maintenance management, impaired
Knowledge deficit (specify)
Mobility, impaired physical

Diagnosis Related Groups

Potentially applicable within all diagnosis related groups

SELF-CONCEPT, DISTURBANCE IN

Nursing Diagnosis

Potential Clinical Findings

Avoidance behaviors
Social isolation
Self-deprecating verbalizations
Lack of eye contact
Stooped posture
Flat or troubled affect
Absent body part(s)
Shame
Anorexic behaviors
Alteration in significant role(s) (recent or unresolved)

Expected Outcomes

The patient will have an increased self-concept.

Interventions

- Identify with the patient

  - sources of threats to self-concept (e.g., altered body image, change in significant roles)
  - coping skills and abilities

- Identify internal and external resources of support systems

  - satisfaction with relationships
  - how decisions are made, by whom
  - hierarchy (who sets limits, who helps with what tasks)
  - marital stability
  - communication patterns
  - relationship with extended family
  - religious beliefs and practices
  - ability to organize after a crisis
  - adaptation to organization and management of daily schedule changes
  - sacrifices necessary for family function and concomitant feelings
  - expectations of others

- financial, educational, and cultural status
- basic physical resources (home, health care, crisis prevention, equipment needs, clothing and food)

- Listen to the patient's expressed feelings; accept their validity.
- Identify signs of grieving and discuss meaning of change and loss.
- Reduce actual or perceived threats as much as possible (specify).
- Introduce changes one at a time; allow adequate adjustment time to avoid threatening the patient's self-concept even further.
- Work with patient to identify personal strengths and potentials.
- Contract with patient to use self-affirmation techniques (e.g., state what "I can" do instead of what "I can't," substitute positive body-image statements for negative ones)
- Evaluate patient's decision-making abilities; provide opportunity for patient to explore alternatives and the consequences of each one.
- Assign/encourage tasks suited to the patient's abilities and limitations; ensure they are ones at which the patient can achieve a degree of success.
- Recognize and praise all efforts in assuming responsibility.
- Consult with other health care professionals (e.g., psychiatric nurse); support their interventions.
- Refer to community support groups as needed; encourage patient to follow up with visits.

Outcome Criteria	The patient has an increased self-concept as evidenced by verbalizations of self-praise; relaxed, appropriate affect and posture; verbalization of personal strengths; and active participation in decision making and completion of tasks.
Potentially Related Nursing Diagnoses	Coping, ineffective individual/family Family process, alteration in Social isolation Thought processes, alteration in
Diagnosis Related Groups	Potentially applicable within all diagnosis related groups

SENSORY-PERCEPTUAL ALTERATION

Nursing Diagnosis

Potential Clinical Findings

Altered sleep pattern
Disorientation
Anxiety
Fear
Hallucinations (e.g., visual, auditory, tactile)
Irritability
Pain
Decreased ability to problem solve
Restlessness
Impaired communication
Frequent, multiple sensory stimuli
Impaired ability to process stimuli
Inappropriate response to stimuli
Invasion of privacy and personal space
Impaired sensory organs
Unfamiliar routines and care givers
Decreased concentration
Impaired mobility
Prolonged confinement in a small area (e.g., private room, ICU)

Expected Outcomes

- The patient will be able to appropriately interpret incoming stimuli.
- The patient will be oriented to person, place, and time.

Interventions

- Identify the source, extent, and implications of the alteration.
- Reduce stimuli as much as possible.
- Provide a quiet atmosphere.
- Identify with the patient sources and functions of incoming stimuli (e.g., "beeps," monitors).
- Provide accurate, factual information; explain all procedures and equipment.

- Place call system and personal articles within easy reach of the patient.
- Monitor vital signs, neurologic status, sleep/activity pattern, responses to stimuli (behavioral and verbalizations).
- Monitor lab results and report significant values
    - ABGs
    - serum drug levels
    - CBC
    - electrolytes
    - chem profile
    - toxicology screen
    - UA
- Reorient patient when necessary; use familiar items
    - personal belongings
    - pictures
    - calendars
    - newspapers
    - television
    - radio
    - clock
- Maintain continuity of care.
- Change patient's room (if possible) if prolonged confinement is contributing to alterations.
- Provide an interpreter as necessary.
- Anticipate patient needs.
- Assist with ADL as necessary.
- Alternate rest periods with nursing care.
- Allow patient to participate in tasks within own capability.
- Involve family/significant others in patient care.
- Identify and reinforce patient's realistic perceptions (e.g., conversation, behavior, concentration).

- Provide opportunity for and assist patient to participate in problem solving within capability.
- Teach patient to compensate for sensory problems (e.g., visual disturbances, right-sided neglect, hearing loss).
- Provide adaptive equipment as needed (e.g., hearing aids, gloves).
- Monitor effectiveness/side effects of prescribed medications.
- Protect patient from injury.
- Consult with other health care professionals (specify).

Outcome Criteria

The patient maintains realistic sensory perceptions as evidenced by appropriate conversation and behavior, verbalized identification of incoming stimuli, increased ability to concentrate and problem solve, and decreased irritability.

Potentially Related Nursing Diagnoses

Coping, ineffective individual
Diversional activity, deficit
Knowledge deficit (specify)
Thought processes, alteration in

Diagnosis Related Groups

Potentially applicable within all diagnosis related groups

Nursing Diagnosis   # SEXUAL DYSFUNCTION

Potential Clinical Findings

Poor body image
Fear
Anxiety
Guilt
Stress
Dissatisfaction
Premature ejaculation
Impotency
Sexual incompatability between partners
Knowledge deficit
Impaired cardiac status
Diabetes
Hypertension
Dyspareunia
Impaired respiratory status

Expected Outcomes

- The patient will identify the sexual dysfunction and its consequences.
- The patient will identify ways to compensate for or resolve the dysfunction.

Interventions

- Assess the source, extent, and implications of the dysfunction.
- Assist patient to express feelings and frustrations regarding the dysfunction; listen therapeutically.
- Avoid judgmental responses to patient.
- Reduce actual/perceived threats as much as possible.
- Help patient to explore sources of stress and anxiety.
- Be reassuring, yet honest.
- Promote patient's self-esteem (e.g., work with patient to identify strengths, reinforce positive attributes).

- Evaluate medications for side effects interfering with sexual function.
- Review "normal" anatomy and physiology with patient.
- Teach patient about any pathophysiology that may be contributing to sexual dysfunction.
- Provide information about alternative means of sexual expression; include the sexual partner in teaching, therapy, etc.
- Teach patient about prescribed medications and the importance of maintaining regimen.
- Refer to other members of the health care team as appropriate (e.g., sex therapist, cardiac rehabilitation nurse).

Outcome Criteria

The patient verbalizes understanding of the dysfunction and methods to compensate for or resolve the dysfunction.

Potentially Related Nursing Diagnoses

Coping, ineffective individual
Coping, ineffective family: compromised
Family process, alteration in
Knowledge deficit (specify)

Diagnosis Related Groups

- Diseases and Disorders of the Nervous System (e.g., spinal disorders and injuries, degenerative nervous system disorders)
- Diseases and Disorders of the Male Reproductive System (e.g., penis procedures, inflammation of the male reproductive system)
- Diseases and Disorders of the Female Reproductive System (e.g., vagina, cervix, and vulva procedures;

infections of the female reproductive system)

- Mental Diseases and Disorders (e.g., acute adjustment reactions and disturbances of psychosocial dysfunction, disorders of personality and impulse control)
- Diseases and Disorders of the Circulatory System (e.g., hypertension, angina pectoris)
- Diseases and Disorders of the Respiratory System (e.g., chronic obstructive pulmonary disease, respiratory neoplasms)
- Diseases and Disorders of the Kidney and Urinary Tract (e.g., renal failure with dialysis; kidney, ureter, and major bladder procedures)
- Myeloproliferative Diseases and Disorders, Poorly Differentiated Malignancy and other Neoplasms (e.g., radiotherapy, chemotherapy)

SKIN INTEGRITY, IMPAIRMENT OF: ACTUAL

Nursing Diagnosis

Potential Clinical Findings

Open lesions
Breakdown
Erythema
Cyanosis
Excretion
Fever
Altered nutritional status
Surgical wounds
Poor personal hygiene
Impaired circulation
Impaired mobility
Altered immune system
Dehydration

Expected Outcomes

- The patient will have warm, dry, intact skin.
- The patient will have formation of granulation tissue in and around the wound.

Interventions

- Assess the source, location, and extent of the impairment.
- Review previous treatments, both helpful and detrimental ones.
- Monitor
  - vital signs (for indications of infection)
  - appearance and characteristics of open areas
  - skin turgor and condition
  - pressure points, bony prominences
  - lab results; report significant values
    * CBC
    * chem profile
    * cultures

- Follow facility protocol for drair
  wounds (i.e., maintain skin a
  wound isolation until cultures a
  negative).
- Institute facility protocol for classifi
  cation and treatment of decubiti and
  burns.
- Teach proper disposal of drainage,
  wastes, dressings, etc.
- Perform incision care as ordered.
- Evaluate effects of creams, oint-
  ments, soaks, and sprays.
- Maintain aseptic technique during
  dressing changes.
- Protect from further impairment
  - utilize alternating pressure mat-
    tresses, egg-crate foam, etc.
  - use sheepskin, skin protectors,
    joint protectors, etc.
  - turn and reposition the patient ev-
    ery 2 hours, alternating pressure
    points
  - provide range of motion to all
    joints
- Maintain nutritional support
  - provide a diet with adequate pro-
    tein and calories
  - ensure adequate fluid intake
- Encourage mobility; get patient out
  of bed on a regular basis.
- Evaluate effectiveness of pain medication.
- Teach patient and care giver techniques to maintain a healthy, intact
  skin.
- Teach patient about prescribed
  medications and the importance of
  maintaining regimen.

Outcome Criteria

The patient regains skin integrity as evidenced by warm, dry intact skin; formation of granulation tissue in and around the breakdown area; and verbalization of increased physical comfort.

Potentially Related Nursing Diagnoses

Comfort, alteration in: pain
Mobility, impaired physical
Tissue perfusion, alteration in

Diagnosis Related Groups

- Diseases and Disorders of the Circulatory System (e.g., atherosclerosis, major reconstructive vascular procedures)
- Diseases and Disorders of the Respiratory System (e.g., interstitial lung disease; OR procedures of the respiratory system)
- Diseases and Disorders of the Kidney and Urinary Tract (e.g., kidney, ureter, and major bladder procedures; renal failure)
- Endocrine, Nutritional, and Metabolic Diseases and Disorders (e.g., diabetes, OR procedures for obesity)
- Diseases and Disorders of the Musculoskeletal System and Connective Tissues (e.g., hip and femur procedures, wound debridement and skin graft)
- Diseases and Disorders of the Digestive System (e.g., inflammatory bowel diseases, rectal resection)
- Diseases and Disorders of the Skin, Subcutaneous Tissue, and Breast (e.g., skin grafts, skin ulcers or cellulitis, subtotal mastectomy)

- Myeloproliferative Diseases and Disorders, Poorly Differentiated Malignancy and other Neoplasms (e.g., chemotherapy, myeloproliferative disorder or poorly differentiated neoplasm with major OR procedure)
- Burns

SKIN INTEGRITY, IMPAIRMENT OF: POTENTIAL

Potential Clinical Findings

Diaphoresis
Poor nutrition
Incontinence
Poor personal hygiene
Impaired mobility
Muscle atrophy
Underweight
Impaired circulation
Fever
Depression
Dehydration
Radiotherapy
Steroid therapy
Allergic reaction
Altered immune system

Expected Outcomes

- The patient's skin will remain warm, dry, intact.
- The patient will demonstrate techniques to maintain skin integrity.

Interventions

- Assess

  - skin turgor and integrity
  - pressure points, bony prominences

- Prevent impairment

  - utilize alternating pressure mattresses, egg-crate foam, as patient's condition indicates
  - use sheepskin, skin protectors, joint protectors, etc.
  - provide range of motion to all joints
  - turn and reposition patient every 2 hours, alternating pressure points

- Maintain nutritional support

- give a diet with adequate protein and calories
- ensure an adequate fluid intake
- Encourage mobility; get the patient out of bed on a regular basis.
- Rub lotions and creams on high-risk areas.
- Teach patient and/or family techniques to maintain an intact skin (e.g., cleanliness; changing position frequently; increasing mobility, nutrition, use of lotions).
- Provide opportunity for and assist patient/family to demonstrate measures to prevent skin breakdown.
- Teach patient about prescribed medications and the importance of maintaining regimen.

Outcome Criteria

- The patient maintains healthy skin as evidenced by a lack of redness or breakdown and verbalization of physical comfort.
- The patient verbalizes and demonstrates active participation in preventing skin breakdown (e.g., foot care, repositioning, applying lotion).

Potentially Related Nursing Diagnoses

Bowel elimination, alteration in: diarrhea/incontinence
Mobility, impaired physical
Self-care deficit (specify level)
Tissue perfusion, alteration in

Diagnosis Related Groups

- Diseases and Disorders of the Nervous System (e.g., spinal disorders and injuries, multiple sclerosis and cerebellar ataxia)

- Diseases and Disorders of the the Circulatory System (e.g., peripheral vascular disorders, circulatory disorders with AMI and cardiovascular compromise)
- Diseases and Disorders of the Respiratory System (e.g., interstitial lung disease, chronic obstructive lung disease)
- Diseases and Disorders of the Kidney and Urinary Tract (e.g., transurethral procedures, kidney and urinary tract infections)
- Endocrine, Nutritional, and Metabolic Diseases and Disorders (e.g., diabetes, inborn errors of metabolism)
- Diseases and Disorders of the Musculoskeletal System and Connective Tissues (e.g., connective tissue disorders, medical back problems)
- Diseases and Disorders of the Digestive System (e.g., inflammatory bowel disorder; esophagitis, gastroenteritis and miscellaneous digestive disorders)
- Diseases and Disorders of the Skin, Subcutaneous Tissue, and Breast (e.g., cellulitis, minor skin disorders)

SLEEP PATTERN DISTURBANCE

Nursing Diagnosis

Potential Clinical Findings

Verbalized lack of sleep
Fatigue
Lethargy
Irritability
Decreased alertness
Increased anxiety
Nausea
Pain
Verbalized interruption of sleep pattern
Tired affect
Slowed verbal responses

Expected Outcomes

The patient will establish an effective sleep pattern.

Interventions

- Take a sleep-activity history, including desired amount of uninterrupted sleep.
- Assess the source of disturbance.
- Listen; understand patient's feelings, frustrations, problems.
- Review patient's use of home sleep aids and their effectiveness.
- Create a relaxing environment with lights and temperature according to patient's preferences.
- Provide emotional support; reassure patient with factual information.
- Provide opportunity for daily physical exercise within patient's capability.
- Place in position of comfort.
- Teach relaxation techniques (e.g., self-hypnosis, biofeedback, "tense and relax").
- Maintain existing bedtime rituals (e.g., snack, prayer, drink, bath).

- Discourage intake of stimulants (e.g., coffee, chocolate) prior to rest period.
- Provide back rub (if desired) before sleep.
- Evaluate effectiveness of prescribed medications.
- Monitor patient when sleeping; particularly note any periods of sleep apnea.
- Allow uninterrupted rest periods.
- Teach patient about prescribed medications and the importance of maintaining regimen.

Outcome Criteria

The patient has established an effective sleep pattern as evidenced by verbalized satisfaction with the sleep pattern; relaxed, cheerful affect; verbalized reduced fatigue; and extended periods of sleep (specify length of uninterrupted sleep).

Potentially Related Nursing Diagnoses

All diagnoses

Diagnosis Related Groups

Potentially applicable within all diagnosis related groups

Nursing Diagnosis	# SOCIAL ISOLATION

Potential Clinical Findings

Lack of contact with others
Withdrawal from family activities
Antisocial behavior
Depression
Altered body image
Fear
Anger
Verbalizes blame on others for own shortcomings
Inability to form significant relationships with others
Inability to meet commitments
Impaired mobility
Loss of significant roles
Loss of significant others
Substance abuse

Expected Outcomes

- The patient will interact with staff and visitors.
- The patient will initiate social contacts and utilize them to meet socialization needs.

Interventions

- Assess

  - perceptions of self, feelings, thoughts, unmet needs, behavior
  - strengths and potentials
  - physical appearance and mental status

- Identify resources for socialization

  - satisfaction with relationships
  - communication patterns
  - relationship with extended family
  - religious beliefs and practices
  - ability to organize after a crisis
  - adaptation to organization and management of daily schedule changes

- financial, educational, and cultural status
  - basic physical resources (home, health care, crisis prevention, clothing and food, transportation)
  - community interaction
  - availability of family and friends
- Identify patient's interests.
- Reduce environmental stress (e.g., open curtains, decrease noise, explain rationale for infection-control measures such as isolation).
- Spend time with patient; communicate acceptance and show genuine interest.
- Promote communication and contact with others (e.g., provide telephone, allow uninterrupted visits with others, put in dayroom).
- Identify and promote interaction between patient and a support person (e.g., relation, friend).
- Explore patient's perceptions of others' behavior.
- Identify with patient's antisocial behaviors.
- Explore with patient alternative social behaviors; teach patient to evaluate consequences of each.
- Help patient to identify and to utilize available coping skills.
- Contract with patient for achievement of a realistic level of social interaction (specify).

Outcome Criteria The patient has increased socialization as evidenced by initiating interaction with staff and visitors; verbalized increased satisfaction with socialization.

Potentially Related Nursing Diagnoses

Coping, ineffective family: compromised
Coping, ineffective individual
Fear
Self-concept, disturbance in
Thought processes, alteration in

Diagnosis Related Groups

- Diseases and Disorders of the Nervous System (e.g., transient ischemic attacks, multiple sclerosis, and cerebellar ataxia)
- Diseases and Disorders of the Respiratory System (e.g., respiratory infections and inflammations, bronchitis and asthma)
- Diseases and Disorders of the Circulatory System (e.g., heart transplant, amputation for circulatory system disorders)
- Diseases and Disorders of the Musculoskeletal System and Connective Tissues (e.g., medical back problems, septic arthritis)
- Endocrine, Nutritional, and Metabolic Diseases and Disorders (e.g., inborn errors of metabolism, skin grafts)
- Myeloproliferative Diseases and Disorders, Poorly Differentiated Malignancy and Other Neoplasms (e.g., lymphoma or leukemia, radiotherapy)
- Mental Diseases and Disorders (e.g., psychoses, depressive neuroses)
- Factors Influencing Health Status and Other Contacts with Health Services (e.g., rehabilitation, other factors influencing health status)

- Substance Use and Induced, Organic Mental Disorders (e.g., drug dependence, alcohol dependence)

SPIRITUAL DISTRESS (DISTRESS OF THE HUMAN SPIRIT)

Nursing Diagnosis

Potential Clinical Findings

Denial
Withdrawal
Fear
Anger
Apathy
Hostility
Worried affect
Inability to accept love/forgiveness
Restlessness
Questioning own beliefs and values, meaning of life and death, own spirituality
Requesting spiritual assistance
Blaming God
Verbalizing concern at inability to continue religious practices

Expected Outcomes

- The patient will feel safe and accepted.
- The patient will establish resolution of conflict in personal belief and value systems.

Interventions

- Evaluate intensity and source of distress.
- Observe appearance, facial and postural affect, eye contact.
- Stay with patient during a crisis.
- Listen to and accept patient's expressions of feelings and fears.
- Reduce environmental stress and hazards (actual or perceived).
- Speak in slow, soft, modulated voice.
- Avoid making statements of false assurance.
- Provide consistent care.

- Help patient distinguish between grief and guilt, if they are contributing to the distress.
- Identify with patient the consequences of acting out of false guilt.
- Provide uninterrupted time for religious practices (provided they are not harmful to the patient or others); facilitate contact with the minister, priest, chaplain, etc., as desired.
- Encourage supportive relationships between patient and others.

Outcome Criteria

The patient resolves belief and value conflicts as evidenced by a relaxed, open affect and posture; verbalizes hope, self-satisfaction, and feelings of peace regarding own spirituality.

Potentially Related Nursing Diagnoses

All diagnoses

Diagnosis Related Groups

Potentially applicable within all diagnosis related groups

THOUGHT PROCESSES, ALTERATION IN

Nursing Diagnosis

Potential Clinical Findings

Short attention span
Agitation
Confusion
Withdrawal
Disorientation
Climbing out of bed
Impaired ability to problem solve
Pulling out lines, tubes, etc.
Fear
Wandering
Incontinence
Inappropriate interaction
Social isolation

Expected Outcomes

- The patient will be oriented to person, place, and time.
- The patient will function optimally within the environment (specify patient's optimal ability).

Interventions

- Observe appearance, facial and postural affect, eye contact, speech patterns, behavior.
- Do a mental status examination.
- Determine the source of the alteration (organic or inorganic).
- Evaluate patient's motivations and self-image.
- Observe for patterns in confused behavior and identify possible aggravating and alleviating factors (e.g., increases at night, improves with light on).
- Monitor lab results and report significant values

  - ABGs
  - CBC

- chem profile
- electrolytes
- drug levels
- UA

- Listen to patient; promote ventilation of feelings by use of leading statements (e.g., "Tell me what you're feeling right now.").
- Provide a quiet environment.
- Be consistent in all approaches to patient.
- Reorient frequently; use familiar items such as

  - personal belongings
  - pictures
  - calendars
  - newspapers
  - television
  - radio
  - clock

- Encourage use of eye glasses and/or hearing aid as needed.
- Protect patient from injury (if indicated, allow patient adequate time to meet ritualistic needs).
- Monitor effectiveness of prescribed medications.
- Communicate and reinforce directions; use repetition and demonstration as necessary.
- Speak in clear, simple sentences maintaining eye contact; keep voice slow and calm.
- Promote supportive relationships between patient and others; encourage participation of family/care givers in patient's care.
- Provide/allow quiet companionship; encourage patient to interact with staff and visitors.

- Inform patient and family about physiologic alterations (if helpful).
- Give honest reassurance; avoid making statements of false assurance.
- Introduce any new material or changes gradually and in a non-threatening way.
- Promote recreational activities and physical exercise as tolerated.

Outcome Criteria

The patient regains usual thought processes as evidenced by orientation to time, place, and person; increased verbalization of reality-based thinking (specific to the individual) and attention span; and active participation in daily care.

Potentially Related Nursing Diagnoses

All diagnoses

Diagnosis Related Groups

- Diseases and Disorders of the Nervous System (e.g., nervous system neoplasms, cranial and peripheral nerve disorders)
- Mental Diseases and Disorders (e.g., disorders of personality and impulse control, psychoses)
- Substance Use and Induced, Organic Mental Disorders (e.g., drug dependence, alcohol- and substance-induced organic mental syndrome)
- Injury, Poisoning, and Toxic Effects of Drugs (e.g., allergic reactions, toxic effects of drugs)

TISSUE PERFUSION, ALTERATION IN

Nursing Diagnosis

Potential Clinical Findings

Ascites
Cyanosis
Necrotic tissue
Cool, pale extremities
Weak or absent peripheral pulses
Edema
Pain
Erythema
Dependent rubor
Prolonged healing time
Burning sensations
Poor skin turgor
Positive Homan's sign
Inflammation
Hardened vein(s)
Fatigue
Lethargy
Neurologic deficits
Decreased alertness
Oliguria
Invasive lines present

Expected Outcomes

- The patient will exhibit an increase in tissue perfusion to affected area.
- The patient will demonstrate measures to improve tissue perfusion to affected area.

Interventions

- Do physical and neurologic assessment.
- Monitor

  - vital signs
  - activity tolerance
  - signs and symptoms of inflammation
  - pain
  - entrance sites of invasive lines

- intake and output
- hemodynamics (e.g., CVP readings, orthostatic changes in vital signs)
- lab results; report significant values

  * ABGs
  * chem profile
  * CBC
  * differential
  * sed rate
  * electrolytes
  * blood cultures
  * UA
  * coagulation studies

- Place in position of comfort.
- Explain all measures and procedures of care.
- Provide measures of comfort (e.g., foam pads, sheepskin).
- Evaluate effectiveness of prescribed medications and oxygen.
- Provide appropriate fluid and dietary requirements per individual needs.
- Instruct patient about dietary restrictions and therapy.
- Keep all skin areas clean and dry.
- Elevate extremities if indicated.
- Evaluate effectiveness of anti-embolitic appliances if used.
- Evaluate effectiveness of heat therapy to affected area as ordered.
- Maintain a warm environment; prevent patient from getting cold.
- Provide opportunity for and encourage physical activity within patient's capability (e.g., isometrics, ambulation).
- Instruct patient to avoid vasoconstrictive positioning (legs crossed, pillow under knees).

- Teach measures to improve perfusion (e.g., specify individual needs such as positioning, medications, activity).
- Provide opportunity for patient to verbalize and demonstrate measures to maximize perfusion.
- Teach patient about prescribed medications and the importance of maintaining regimen.
- Teach patient about prevention of potential problems of chronic anticoagulation (e.g., need for monitoring blood levels, regular follow-up visits, protect from injury).

Outcome Criteria

- The patient exhibits an increase in tissue perfusion as evidenced by strong peripheral pulses; warm, dry extremities with unimpaired movement and sensation; vital signs within normal limits; appropriate wakefulness, alertness, and orientation; verbalizes increased comfort; absence of edema; balanced intake and output; and even and unlabored respirations.
- The patient verbalizes and demonstrates measures to improve tissue perfusion (specify, e.g., positioning, mobility, diet, antiembolic appliances).

Potentially Related Nursing Diagnoses

Cardiac output, alteration in: decreased
Gas exchange, impaired
Injury, potential for

Diagnosis Related Groups

- Burns
- Diseases and Disorders of the Nervous System (e.g., extracranial

vascular procedures, specific cerebrovascular disorders)

- Diseases and Disorders of Blood and Blood Forming Organs and Immunity Disorders (e.g., coagulation disorders, red blood cell disorders)
- Diseases and Disorders of the Circulatory System (e.g., deep vein thrombophlebitis, peripheral vascular disorders)

URINARY ELIMINATION, ALTERATION IN PATTERNS

Nursing Diagnosis

Potential Clinical Findings

Foul, dark urine
Cloudy urine
Dysuria
Incontinence
Frequent, small voidings
Oliguria
Polyuria
Distended bladder
Inability to void
Dehydration
Constipation
Recent anesthesia
Use of narcotic analgesics
Hematuria
Decreased bladder sensation
Urinary catheter in place

Expected Outcomes

- The patient will be continent at all times.
- The patient will empty bladder with every voiding.

Interventions

- Do an abdominal assessment with digital rectal exam, unless otherwise indicated.
- Monitor

  - intake and output
  - vital signs (orthostatic changes)
  - bladder distention (palpate bladder gently)
  - characteristics of urine (color, amount, odor)
  - voiding frequency
  - skin turgor and integrity
  - pain
  - lab results; report significant values

* UA
  * occult blood
  * urine pH and specific gravity
  * urine glucose and acetone
  * urine electrolytes
  * urine C&S
  * 24-hour creatinine clearance
  * CBC
  * diff
  * sed rate
  * chem profile
  * electrolytes

  - breath sounds
  - edema
  - neck vein distention
  - changes in level of consciousness

- Allow a regular opportunity to void; do not rush the patient, assist with sitting/standing if necessary.
- Facilitate voiding (e.g., utilize sitz bath, warm water over perineum, running water, privacy) as needed.
- Monitor effectiveness of prescribed medications.
- Evaluate results of catheterization.
- Maintain consistent perineal hygiene.
- Work with patient to ensure adherence to prescribed fluid restriction or excess.
- Evaluate oral mucosa and give oral hygiene as needed.
- Instruct patient to respond rapidly to urge to void.
- Instruct patient in bladder regimen (specify to individual needs, e.g., offer assistance to void every 2-4 hours; self-catheterization).
- Provide opportunity for patient to verbalize and demonstrate compre-

hension of prescribed bladder regimen.
- Teach patient about prescribed medications and importance of maintaining regimen.
- Consult with other members of the health care team (specify) as necessary.

Outcome Criteria

The patient has established an effective pattern of urinary elimination as evidenced by continence, voiding sufficient quantity (specify per individual), bladder not palpable after voiding, and significant lab values within normal limits; verbalizes comfort and satisfaction with voiding pattern.

Potentially Related Nursing Diagnoses

Health maintenance, alteration in
Home maintenance management, impaired
Fluid volume deficit, actual or potential
Self-care deficit (specify level)

Diagnosis Related Groups

- Diseases and Disorders of the Nervous System (e.g., spinal disorders and injuries, multiple sclerosis, and cerebellar ataxia)
- Diseases and Disorders of the Circulatory System (e.g., heart failure and shock, hypertension)
- Endocrine, Nutritional, and Metabolic Diseases and Disorders (e.g., diabetes, endocrine disorders)
- Diseases and Disorders of the Kidney and Urinary Tract (e.g., urethral procedures, urinary stones)
- Diseases and Disorders of the Male Reproductive System (e.g., benign prostatic hypertrophy, penis procedures)

- Diseases and Disorders of the Female Reproductive System (e.g., female reproductive system reconstructive procedures; vagina, cervix, and vulva procedures)
- Pregnancy, Childbirth, and the Puerperium (e.g., cesarean section, vaginal delivery)
- Myeloproliferative Diseases and Disorders, Poorly Differentiated Malignancy and Other Neoplasms (e.g., radiotherapy, chemotherapy)

VIOLENCE, POTENTIAL FOR

Potential Clinical Findings

Aggressive behavior
Paranoid behavior
Anger
Fear
Depression
Ambivalence
Hallucinations
Verbalization of threats
Social isolation
Tense, rigid posture
Substance abuse
Clenched fists
Increased motor activity
Threatening gestures
Presence of a weapon

Expected Outcomes

- The patient will behave in a nonviolent manner.
- The patient will maintain self-control.

Interventions

- Observe
    - physical posture and expression
    - verbal and nonverbal behavior
    - interactions with family and friends

- Listen to and evaluate reported observations of patient's behavior.
- Identify aggravating and alleviating factors that could lead to violent behavior in this patient.
- Acknowledge staff's intuitive feelings of fear and danger.
- Take threats of violence seriously.
- Protect others.
- Reduce environmental noise, distraction, stimulation; ensure privacy.
- Call patient by name.

- Use a calm, reassuring voice and manner.
- Maintain distance from patient (touch may cause loss of control).
- Do not make threats to patient; clearly state limits and consequences of unacceptable behavior, and enforce the consequences when the limits have been exceeded.
- Avoid creating a power struggle; be consistent and firm in all interactions with patient.
- Help the patient identify
  - early signs of losing control
  - inappropriate behavior
  - consequences of violent behavior (including harm to self)
  - alternative expressions of negative feelings
- Teach patient that it is all right to experience all emotions but the resulting behavior must be appropriate.
- Encourage patient to identify and discuss feelings about any incident that precipitates loss of control.
- Verbally acknowledge the patient's feelings as valid (e.g., "I'm sure you feel angry right now.").
- Reinforce all appropriate behavior.
- Do not leave the patient alone when exhibiting violent tendencies to self.
- Give clear, direct commands to assist patient in gaining self-control.
- Consult other members of the health care team as needed.
- Refer patient to community resources and encourage to follow through with appointments.

Outcome Criteria	The patient maintains nonviolent self-control as evidenced by no harm to self or others, active selection and use of nonviolent appropriate means of expression, verbalized feelings of self-control, and relaxed affect and posture.

Potentially Related Nursing Diagnoses

Fear
Grieving, dysfuntional
Thought processes, alterations in

Diagnosis Related Groups

- Diseases and Disorders of the Nervous System (e.g., craniotomy, concussion)
- Mental Diseases and Disorders (e.g., psychoses, disorders of personality and impulse control)
- Substance Use and Induced, Organic Mental Disorders (e.g., alcohol- and substance-induced organic mental syndrome, drug dependence)
- Injury, Poisoning, and Toxic Effects of Drugs (e.g., allergic reactions, toxic effects of drugs)

Abbreviations

ABGs	arterial blood gases
ADL	activities of daily living
AFB	acid-fast bacilli
AMI	acute myocardial infarct
BUN	blood urea nitrogen
C&S	culture and sensitivities
CBC	complete blood count
chem profile	chemistry profile
diff	differential
ECG	electrocardiograph
npo	nothing by mouth
PT	prothrombin time
PTT	partial thromboplastin time
sed rate	sedimentation rate
UA	urinalysis

**Nursing Diagnoses Potentially
Applicable Within all Diagnosis
Related Groups**

Anxiety
Comfort, Alteration in: Pain
Coping, Family: Potential For
Growth
Coping, Ineffective Family:
Compromised
Coping, Ineffective Family:
Disabling
Coping, Ineffective Individual
Diversional Activity, Deficit
Family Process, Alteration in
Fear
Grieving, Anticipatory
Grieving, Dysfunctional
Health Maintenance, Alteration in
Home Maintenance Management,
Impaired
Knowledge Deficit (specify)
Noncompliance (specify)
Oral Mucous Membrane,
Alteration in
Powerlessness
Self-Care Deficit (specify level)
Self-Concept, Disturbance in
Sensory-Perceptual Alteration
Sleep Pattern Disturbance
Spiritual Distress (Distress of the
Human Spirit)

**Diseases and Disorders of Blood and
Blood Forming Organs and Immunity
Disorders**

Injury, Potential for
Nutrition, Alteration in: Less Than
Body Requirements
Tissue Perfusion, Alteration in

Burns

Fluid Volume Deficit, Actual or Potential

Nutrition, Alteration in: Less Than Body Requirements

Skin Integrity, Impairment of: Actual

Tissue Perfusion, Alteration in

Diseases and Disorders of the Circulatory System

Activity Intolerance, Actual or Potential

Airway Clearance, Ineffective

Bowel Elimination, Alteration in: Constipation

Breathing Pattern, Ineffective

Cardiac Output, Alteration in: Decreased

Communication, Impaired: Verbal

Fluid Volume, Alteration in: Excess

Fluid Volume Deficit, Actual or Potential

Gas Exchange, Impaired

Injury, Potential for

Mobility, Impaired Physical

Nutrition, Alteration in: Less Than Body Requirements

Nutrition, Alteration in: Potential for More than Body Requirements

Sexual Dysfunction

Skin Integrity, Impairment of: Actual

Skin Integrity, Impairment of: Potential

Social Isolation

Tissue Perfusion, Alteration in

Urinary Elimination, Alteration in Patterns

Diseases and Disorders of the Digestive System

Activity Intolerance, Actual or Potential

Bowel Elimination, Alteration in: Constipation

Bowel Elimination, Alteration in: Diarrhea

Bowel Elimination, Alteration in: Incontinence

Fluid Volume, Alteration in: Excess

Fluid Volume Deficit, Actual or Potential

Gas Exchange, Impaired

Injury, Potential for

Mobility, Impaired Physical

Nutrition, Alteration in: Less Than Body Requirements

Nutrition, Alteration in: Potential for More than Body Requirements

Oral Mucous Membrane, Alteration in

Skin Integrity, Impairment of: Actual

Skin Integrity, Impairment of: Potential

Tissue Perfusion: Alteration in

Diseases and Disorders of the Ear, Nose, and Throat

Activity Intolerance, Actual or Potential

Airway Clearance, Ineffective

Breathing Pattern, Ineffective

Communication, Impaired: Verbal

Injury, Potential for

Mobility, Impaired Physical

Nutrition, Alteration in: Less Than Body Requirements

Sensory-Perceptual Alteration

Endocrine, Nutritional, and Metabolic Diseases and Disorders

Bowel Elimination, Alteration in: Diarrhea
Fluid Volume, Alteration in: Excess
Gas Exchange, Impaired
Injury, Potential for
Nutrition, Alteration in: Less Than Body Requirements
Nutrition, Alteration in: More Than Body Requirements
Nutrition, Alteration in: Potential for More than Body Requirements
Skin Integrity, Impairment of: Actual
Skin Integrity, Impairment of: Potential
Social Isolation
Urinary Elimination, Alteration in Patterns

Diseases and Disorders of the Eye

Injury, Potential for
Mobility, Impaired Physical
Sensory-Perceptual Alteration

Diseases and Disorders of the Hepatobiliary System and Pancreas

Bowel Elimination, Alteration in: Diarrhea
Fluid Volume, Alteration in: Excess
Injury, Potential for
Nutrition, Alteration in: Less Than Body Requirements
Nutrition, Alteration in: Potential for More than Body Requirements

Factors Influencing Health Status and Other Contacts with Health Services

Coping, Ineffective Individual
Health Maintenance, Alteration in
Knowledge Deficit

Noncompliance
Social Isolation

**Diseases and Disorders of the Female
Reproductive System**
Injury, Potential for
Rape-Trauma Syndrome
Sexual Dysfunction
Urinary Elimination, Alteration in
Patterns

Infectious and Parasitic Diseases
Bowel Elimination, Alteration in:
Diarrhea
Gas Exchange, Impaired
Injury, Potential for
Nutrition, Alteration in: Less Than
Body Requirements

**Injury, Poisoning, and Toxic Effects of
Drugs**
Gas Exchange, Impaired
Injury, Potential for
Thought Processes, Alteration in
Violence, Potential for

**Diseases and Disorders of the Kidney
and Urinary Tract**
Fluid Volume, Alteration in: Excess
Fluid Volume Deficit, Actual or
Potential
Injury, Potential for
Nutrition, Alteration in: Potential for
More than Body Requirements
Rape-Trauma Syndrome
Sexual Dysfunction
Skin Integrity, Impairment of:
Actual
Skin Integrity, Impairment of:
Potential
Tissue Perfusion, Alteration in
Urinary Elimination, Alteration in
Patterns

Diseases and Disorders of the Male Reproductive System
Injury, Potential for
Rape-Trauma Syndrome
Sexual Dysfunction
Urinary Elimination, Alteration in Patterns

Mental Diseases and Disorders
Injury, Potential for
Nutrition, Alteration in: Less Than Body Requirements
Nutrition, Alteration in: More Than Body Requirements
Nutrition, Alteration in: Potential for More than Body Requirements
Parenting, Alteration in: Actual or Potential
Rape-Trauma Syndrome
Sexual Dysfunction
Social Isolation
Thought Processes, Alteration in
Violence, Potential For

Diseases and Disorders of the Musculoskeletal System and Connective Tissues
Activity Intolerance, Actual or Potential
Fluid Volume, Alteration in: Excess
Gas Exchange, Impaired
Injury, Potential for
Mobility, Impaired Physical
Skin Integrity, Impairment of: Actual
Skin Integrity, Impairment of: Potential
Social Isolation

Myeloproliferative Diseases and Disorders, Poorly Differentiated Malignancy and other Neoplasms

Gas Exchange, Impaired
Injury, Potential for
Nutrition, Alteration in: Less Than Body Requirements
Sexual Dysfunction
Skin Integrity, Impairment of: Actual
Social Isolation
Urinary Elimination, Alteration in Patterns

Diseases and Disorders of the Nervous System

Activity Intolerance, Actual or Potential
Airway Clearance, Ineffective
Bowel Elimination, Alteration in: Constipation
Bowel Elimination, Alteration in: Incontinence
Breathing Pattern, Ineffective
Communication, Impaired: Verbal
Fluid Volume, Alteration in: Excess
Gas Exchange, Impaired
Injury, Potential for
Mobility, Impaired Physical
Nutrition, Alteration in: Less Than Body Requirements
Sensory-Perceptual Alteration
Sexual Dysfunction
Skin Integrity, Impairment of: Potential
Social Isolation
Thought Processes, Alteration in
Tissue Perfusion, Alteration in
Urinary Elimination, Alteration in Patterns
Violence, Potential For

Newborns and other Neonates with Conditions Originating in the Perinatal Period
Bowel Elimination, Alteration in: Diarrhea
Injury, Potential for
Nutrition, Alteration in: Less Than Body Requirements
Parenting, Alteration in: Actual or Potential

Pregnancy, Childbirth, and the Puerperium
Nutrition, Alteration in: Less Than Body Requirements
Nutrition, Alteration in: Potential for More than Body Requirements
Parenting, Alteration in: Actual or Potential
Urinary Elimination, Alteration in Patterns

Diseases and Disorders of the Respiratory System
Activity Intolerance, Actual or Potential
Airway Clearance, Ineffective
Bowel Elimination, Alteration in: Constipation
Breathing Pattern, Ineffective
Cardiac Output, Alteration in: Decreased
Communication, Impaired: Verbal
Fluid Volume, Alteration in: Excess
Fluid Volume Deficit, Actual or Potential
Gas Exchange, Impaired
Injury, Potential for
Mobility, Impaired Physical
Nutrition, Alteration in: Less Than Body Requirements
Sexual Dysfunction

Skin Integrity, Impairment of:
Actual
Skin Integrity, Impairment of:
Potential
Social Isolation

**Diseases and Disorders of the Skin,
Subcutaneous Tissue, and Breast**
Skin Integrity, Impairment of:
Actual
Skin Integrity, Impairment of:
Potential
Tissue Perfusion, Alteration in

**Substance Use and Induced, Organic
Mental Disorders**
Gas Exchange, Impaired
Nutrition, Alteration in: Less Than
Body Requirements
Social Isolation
Thought Processes, Alteration in
Violence, Potential For

Sample Nursing Care Plans

The following examples include brief case histories and individualized nursing care plans. The patients are fictitious and any resemblance to actual persons is coincidental. It is recognized that treatment protocols vary from region to region; however, care plans should reflect accepted standards of care in each facility. Also, target dates should represent the diagnosis related group projected length of stay for each patient. It is assumed that care plans must be updated throughout the patient's course of service, and must reflect the patient's readiness for discharge.

JANE MARBLE   Admitting Diagnosis: PNEUMONIA

History Present Illness

Ms. Marble 2 weeks ago she had "flu symptoms" that resolved except for persistent nasal congestion and sore throat. Last evening she developed sudden onset of "shaking and chills" with fever of 39° C. Fever persisted throughout the night, and early this morning she developed "stabbing chest pain" in the left lower midaxillary region with inspiration. The patient brought herself to the emergency department.

Past Medical History

Essentially negative

Allergies

No known allergies

Physical Examination

Presentation

- Alert and oriented to person, place, and time; responds appropriately
- Speech is slow and monotonous; unable to speak in complete sentences
- Sitting upright in bed, splinting her chest with a pillow. Facial expression is grimacing and tense, and she states, "I can't get a deep enough breath to get in enough air."

Skin

- Pale, hot, and dry with a facial flush

- Turgor: decreased elasticity and slow return

Eyes, Ears, Nose, Throat
- Pupils equal, round, reactive to light
- No drainage
- No ear discomfort
- Nasal passages patent with mucosa dry and intact; nasal flaring with inspiration
- Oral mucous membrane pink and dry, intact; breath malodorous
- Throat red; tonsils present and erythematous
- Cervical lymph nodes palpable and tender

Cardiac
- Blood pressure 110/70, apical pulse 108/minute; regular rate and rhythm without murmur
- Extremities warm and pink; nailbed capillary refill less than 2 seconds

Respiratory
- Respirations rapid and shallow at rate of 40/minute
- Splints chest with a pillow
- Persistent, involuntary cough nonproductive of sputum
- Breath sounds diminished in bases bilaterally; coarse rales in the left middle lobe and a rubbing sound heard in the left lower midaxillary region; complains of pain on inspiration in the area around the rub
- Left mid-lower lobes sound flat to percussion

Gastrointestinal
- Abdomen slightly distended, nontender to palpation
- Active bowel sounds in all quadrants
- Reports intermittent nausea but no vomiting
- Height 5 ft 4 in; weight 120 lb; has had an 8-lb weight loss in the past 2 weeks
- Appetite is decreased; states, "I have no desire for food."

Genitourinary
- Reports infrequent voiding (small amounts of dark-amber urine about 3 times/day) during the past 2 days; denies foul odor of urine
- No pain or burning with urination

| Ineffective airway clearance related to pain | Target date: 7 days 1. Patient's respirations will be even and unlabored. 2. Chest will be clear to auscultation. | 1. Complete chest assessment every shift and prn. 2. Evaluate air exchange every shift and prn; monitor vital signs every 4 hours and prn. 3. Monitor and record amount and characteristics of all sputum. 4. Evaluate lab values; report to MD significant changes in
 – ABGs
 – CBC, sed rate
 – blood cultures
 – sputum C&S, AFB, gram stain
 – chest x-ray
 – ECG
 – intradermal skin tests (e.g., PPD) 5. Place in position of comfort (high/semi-Fowler's). 6. Administer humidified oxygen by nasal cannula at 5 liters/minute and evaluate effectiveness. 7. Evaluate the effectiveness of medications. 8. Assist with chest physical therapy while | 1. Even, unlabored respiration at a rate of 16–20/minute 2. Breath sounds clear to auscultation 3. Increased ease in breathing (confirmed by patient) |

JANE MARBLE Admitting Diagnosis: PNEUMONIA *(continued)*

Nursing Diagnosis	Expected Outcomes	Ongoing Assessment and Interventions	Outcome
		awake; evaluate the effects of nebulizer treatments – perform postural drainage with percussion every 4 hours while awake (follow nebulizer treatments). – instruct and receive return demonstration on turning, coughing, and deep breathing every 2 hours while awake. 9. Maintain a cool patient environment with a constant air flow; use a cool-air humidifier at bedside as ordered.	

Alteration in comfort: pain related to pleural rub and persistent cough	*Target Date:* 7 days
	1. Patient's comfort will increase.
		1. Assess the etiology of the pain
		  – location (with or without radiation)
		  – intensity
		  – duration
		  – aggravating factors
		  – alleviating factors
		  – frequency.
		2. Monitor pt.'s behavior
		  – facial affect
		  – body posturing
		  – tone of voice
		  – activity
		  – speech.
		3. Provide dry heat to back and chest areas prn discomfort.
		4. Listen responsively to verbalizations of discomfort; explain rationale for each intervention.
		5. Coordinate nursing treatments to allow rest periods.
		6. Promote relaxation
		  – reduce noise
		  – place in comfortable position
		  – give back rubs at hs and prn
		  – encourage splinting of chest prn.
		7. Assess effectiveness of pain medications.
			1. Decreased intensity of discomfort (confirmed by patient)
			2. More relaxed affect
			3. Greater ease of movement; less need to splint the chest

JANE MARBLE   Admitting Diagnosis: PNEUMONIA *(continued)*

Nursing Diagnosis	Expected Outcomes	Ongoing Assessment and Interventions	Outcome
Fear related to hospitalization and shortness of breath	*Target Date:* 24 hours 1. Patient will identify fear-producing perceptions and will participate in steps to alleviate any misconceptions.	1. Explain procedures, medications, and treatments in advance. 2. Discuss thoughts about hospitalization; correct any misconceptions. 3. Provide continuity in nursing care. 4. Foster realistic expectations of improved health with time and treatment. 5. Teach pt. to use the call system; keep it readily available and answer light promptly.	1. Verbalizes fear-producing perceptions 2. Attention to explanations of care 3. Less fear, increased relaxation, feelings of ease (confirmed by patient)
Fluid volume deficit related to fever, increased metabolic rate, and decreased intake	*Target Date:* 2 days 1. Patient will return to a state of fluid balance.	1. Monitor – I&O (instruct pt.) – urine specific gravity (all urine samples) – orthostatic vital signs bid and prn – lab values (be alert to the fact that dehydration will cause hemoconcentration, increasing some values; report significant changes to MD)	1. Warm, pink, intact skin; elasticity with rapid return 2. Oral mucosa moist and intact 3. Temperature consistently 37.0°–37.2°C

	4. Increased fluid intake (2,000–3,000 cc/24 hours)

– level of consciousness and behavior
  – skin turgor, oral mucosa every shift.
2. Force clear liquids: 1–2 8-oz glasses every 2 hours while awake
  – limit milk products to ½ cup daily
  – avoid excessively hot or cold fluids
  – prefers cranberry juice and lemon-lime soda.
3. Insert and maintain IV as ordered; assess for symptoms of overhydration every shift and prn.
4. Provide oral hygiene every 2–4 hours and prn.
5. Monitor temperature every 2 hours and prn; evaluate effectivess of antipyretic measures.
6. Obtain blood cultures x 2, at different sites or 15 minutes apart, for fever greater than 38.6 C.	

JANE MARBLE   Admitting Diagnosis: PNEUMONIA *(continued)*

Nursing Diagnosis	Expected Outcomes	Ongoing Assessment and Interventions	Outcome

Activity intolerance related to increased shortness of breath and fatigue	*Target Date*: 2 days
	1. Patient demonstrates increased ability to tolerate ADL.
		1. Assess the source, extent, and implications of the activity intolerance every shift and prn.
		
		2. Assist with bathroom privileges and give a bed bath in the first 24 hours after admission.
		
		3. After 24 hours, promote increased participation with ADL (e.g., grooming, bathing, feeding).
		
		4. Promote out-of-bed activity as tolerated, per order
		  – bathroom privileges
		  – up in chair for 30 minutes, at least tid
		  – progressive ambulation.
			1. Requests to take a shower
			
			2. Initiates morning oral care
			
			3. Increased strength and autonomy in grooming, bathing, and feeding (confirmed by patient)

| Alteration in nutrition: less than body requirements related to increased metabolic rate and decreased nutrient intake | Target Date: 5 days
1. Patient will increase nutrient intake to balance diet and meet increased metabolic needs. | 1. Obtain diet history for the past week.
2. Assess food likes and dislikes.
3. Obtain weight (in gown) at the same time every day.
4. Monitor lab values and report significant changes to MD.
5. Provide 6 small feedings daily, including as many preferred foods as possible; be sure pt. understands the rationale for this schedule.
6. Advance diet (from liquid to general) as tolerated, per order.
7. Provide rest periods before, during, and after meals.
8. Medicate for discomfort prn before feedings; evaluate response.
9. Provide attractive meal trays.
10. Avoid excessively hot or cold food.
11. Identify flatus-generating foods; avoid serving them.
12. Consult with dietician to assure high-calorie, high-protein diet; monitor calorie count prn. | 1. Caloric intake of 2,500–3,000 calories daily
2. Increased appetite (confirmed by patient); request for more food at mealtimes
3. Normal lab values
4. Gain of 2 lb since admission |

JESSIE BIRCH	**Home-care Referral for Home Assessment and Self-care Instruction**

Age 73

Medical Problems

Congestive heart failure
Adult-onset diabetes mellitus
Blind in left eye; decreased vision in right eye (secondary to cataract condition)
rheumatoid arthritis with acute exacerbation in left knee

Medications

Furosemide	40 mg po bid
Digoxin	0.125 mg po daily
Chlorpropamide	250 mg po daily
Enteric-coated aspirin	650 mg po bid

Prescribed diet Sodium restricted, 1,500 calorie ADA

Notes from Initial Visit

Mrs. Birch is a widowed, black female and lives alone in a high-rise apartment building for senior citizens. Her apartment is cluttered but not dirty. There are many small throw rugs throughout the apartment. She lives on a small, fixed income. She has no family in the state except an older sister in a nursing home on the other side of the city, with whom Mrs. Birch infrequently visits via telephone. Mrs. Birch is up and dressed when the nurse arrives. (She usually awakens about 9:00 AM and gets up about 9:15 AM; bedtime is around 11:00 PM.) Physical exam reveals clear lungs, regular apical pulse 88/minute, and no cough. There is slight bilateral ankle edema. She is able to read large print with her right eye. Her left knee is edematous and warm, and is painful with manipulation and weight bearing. Mrs. Birch ambulates with a cane and it is very difficult for her to shop, visit, or see the MD because of limited mobility and finances. She voices much chagrin over her lack of socialization.

Mrs. Birch has a large pot of greens boiling on the stove. She states that her diet consists mainly of TV dinners, greens, pork, and vegetables.

Nursing Diagnosis	Expected Outcomes	Ongoing Assessment and Interventions	Outcome
Alteration in cardiac output: decreased related to prior myocardial infarction	*Target Date:* 3rd visit 1. Patient's cardiac output will remain stable. 2. Patient will be able to state signs and symptoms of decreasing cardiac output, and will call nurse when they occur.	1. Monitor vital signs, weight, breath sounds, and edema biweekly until baseline is established and stabilized. 2. Establish appropriate daily medication regimen (with meals) – all morning meds at 10:00 AM. – all evening meds at 8:00 PM. 3. Institute a sodium-restricted diet. 4. Teach pt. to put feet up when sitting and to lie down and rest for 1 hour each afternoon. 5. Instruct pt. to call nurse if signs or symptoms of acute cardiac decompensation occur – marked shortness of breath – marked increase in edema – irregular heart beat – unrelieved dizziness.	1. Stable vital signs 2. No increase in edema

JESSIE BIRCH Home-care Referral for Home Assessment and Self-care Instruction
(continued)

Nursing Diagnosis	Expected Outcomes	Ongoing Assessment and Interventions	Outcome
Potential for injury related to use of cane, decreased mobility, and unsafe environment (multiple loose throw rugs in apartment)	*Target Date:* 3rd visit 1. Patient will remain free from injury. 2. Patient will decrease risk of injury.	1. Assess pt.'s apartment; look for ways to decrease/eliminate obstacles that could cause a fall. 2. Discuss the hazards of throw rugs. Find out what purpose they serve and replace them with safer alternatives (e.g., nonskid appliques on tile flooring) to decrease danger of slipping. 3. Evaluate stability of pt.'s cane-assisted ambulation. 4. Provide necessary adaptive equipment (e.g., 3-prong cane, tongs for reaching and grasping objects, walker).	1. Fewer obstacles in living environment 2. Absence of injury

Alteration in comfort: pain related to joint inflammation	Target Date: 2nd visit
	1. Patient will successfully manage pain at home.
		1. Assess pain each visit
		  – etiology
		  – intensity
		  – frequency
		  – duration
		  – aggravating factors
		  – alleviating factors.
		2. Instruct pt. not to stress painful joints, but to gradually move them through range of motion daily.
		3. Teach appropriate use of heat/cold treatments
		  – use cold treatments (15–20 minutes every 1–2 hours) to relieve red, swollen, warm, painful joints.
		  – apply heat (15–20 minutes every 1–2 hours) to stiff, painful joints that are not red and warm to the touch.
		4. Allow pt. an opportunity to ventilate feelings about pain.
			1. Control of pain by use of learned measures (confirmed by patient)
			2. Appropriate use of heat and cold therapy

JESSIE BIRCH **Home-care Referral for Home Assessment and Self-care Instruction** *(continued)*

Nursing Diagnosis	Expected Outcomes	Ongoing Assessment and Interventions	Outcome
Knowledge deficit regarding salt-restricted and ADA diets Potential noncompliance with dietary regimen related to knowledge deficit	*Target Date:* 5th visit 1. Patient will be able to describe and follow prescribed diet.	1. Notify pt. in advance that you wish to discuss prescribed diet and means of compliance. 2. Have pt. prepare a diet diary for 3 days, and a list of foods that she considers staples. 3. Assess diet diary and review it with pt., ascertaining what foods have particular cultural value. 4. Make a list (in large print) of foods low and high in sodium (be certain to include all the foods the pt. listed). 5. Obtain large-print, illustrated copy of 1,500-calorie ADA diet; mark acceptable foods on the sodium-restricted list. 6. Discuss using Meals-on-Wheels; arrange for delivery of weekday lunches.	

		7. Review the diet list with pt.; help make out menus and shopping lists.	1. Menus and meals follow the prescribed diet
		8. On each visit, reinforce new behavior; help pt. plan menus utilizing foods that are important to her; include foods with high potassium content.	2. Lab work and exams reflect diet compliance (confirmed by patient's MD)
Social isolation related to impaired mobility, limited finances	*Target Date*: 4th visit 1. Patient will initiate social contacts; will develop an ongoing schedule to meet socialization needs.	1. Arrange for senior citizen discount transportation; teach pt. about its use and benefits. 2. Have pt. arrange a time to visit her sister, using the special transportation. 3. Tell pt. about neighborhood "phone friends" organization (shut-in neighbors call a friend several times weekly to chat). 4. Introduce pt. to area senior citizen center; provide schedules of events and shuttle service.	1. Expresses satisfaction with socialization 2. Expresses interest in activities 3. Explores/utilizes social opportunities

MIA PERRIN   Admitting Diagnosis: FULL-TERM PREGNANCY (currently 48 hours postpartum)

History
- Para i, gravida i
- Rh+, rubella titer 1:2
- Labor lasted 12 hours with spontaneous rupture of membranes; uncomplicated vaginal delivery with a midline episiotomy
- Medication taken during pregnancy: prenatal vitamins with iron
- Weight gain with pregnancy: 30 lb (usual weight is 116 lb); height 5 ft 4 in

Physical Examination

Mrs. Perrin is well groomed. Her skin is warm and moist. The oral mucous membranes are pink and moist; there are no lesions present and teeth are in good repair. The lungs are clear to auscultation with even, unlabored respirations at a rate of 16/minute. Oral temperature is 37.1°C. Her breasts are symmetrical, soft, and nontender. The nipples are red and tender. Her abdomen is soft and bowel tones are present in all four quadrants. Her bowel movement this morning was soft; denies difficulty with evacuation. Her fundus is firm and its position is in the midline below the umbilicus after voiding. The lochia is serosa and moderate. The episiotomy incision is clean and intact; slightly reddened and swollen; reports tenderness around the incisional area.

Mrs. Perrin ambulates with a slow, steady gait and has active range of motion in all extremities.

Psychosocial

Mrs. Perrin understands concepts and verbalizes appropriate questions. Her speech is clear (in English) and audible. Direct eye contact is maintained. She is cooperative and concerned about postpartum care of her breasts and episiotomy. She interacts with her infant by cuddling, kissing, and talking, but expresses anxiety about her inexperience with infants and ability to master bathing, cord care, female perineal care, and infant stimulation.

Baby girl Perrin weighs 7 lb 15 oz, is 21 inches long, and nurses on demand, every 2½–3 hours.

JESSIE BIRCH Home-care Referral for Home Assessment and Self-care Instruction (continued)

Nursing Diagnosis	Expected Outcomes	Ongoing Assessment and Interventions	Outcome
Alteration in comfort: pain related to postpartal swelling of episiotomy	*Target Date*: 3 days 1. Patient will have decreased swelling and discomfort in her perineum and episiotomy.	1. Assess episiotomy every 4 hours for – approximation – color – increased swelling – discharge or hardness around the incision. 2. Apply warm wet packs for 1 hour qid and prm to perineum; monitor effectiveness. 3. Apply Xylocaine jelly 2% topically to perineal area after each voiding and prm; monitor effectiveness. 4. Apply heat lamp to perineum 20 minutes tid ar.d prm; monitor effectiveness. 5. Medicate as ordered and monitor effectiveness; if ineffective call MD.	1. Dry, intact perineum and episiotomy; no increase in edema 2. Decreased discomfort (confirmed by patient) 3. Fewer requests for pain medication and prm treatments

MIA PERRIN   Admitting Diagnosis: FULL-TERM PREGNANCY *(continued)*

Nursing Diagnosis	Expected Outcomes	Ongoing Assessment and Interventions	Outcome

Impaired skin integrity (tender, red nipples) related to breast-feeding	*Target Date*: 3 days
	1. Patient's nipples will be less tender.
	2. Skin around nipples will remain intact.
		1. Assess breasts and nipples before each feeding for redness or swelling.
		2. Provide necessary nursing instruction
		  – emphasize the importance of a well-fitting nursing bra.
		  – wash and airdry nipples at least tid; do not dry with a towel.
		  – leave nursing bra flaps open for 30-45 minutes after breast-feedings to allow nipples to air dry.
			1. Decreased reports of discomfort related to breast-feeding
			2. Reduced redness and tenderness around nipples; skin intact

Knowledge deficit regarding general postpartum and newborn care	*Target Date*: 3 days 1. Parents will verbalize and demonstrate general knowledge of postpartum and newborn care.	1. Institute and utilize the facility's standard teaching guidelines. 2. Assess specific learning needs for more in-depth instruction. 3. Provide an environment conducive to learning.	1. Verbal demonstration of accurate general knowledge of postpartum and newborn care

2. Parents will verbalize and demonstrate knowledge of infant bathing, cord care, and infant (female) perineal care.	4. Include both parents in teaching sessions whenever possible.
	5. Utilize written/spoken demonstration and return-demonstration teaching techniques.
	6. Instruct on infant bathing
	  – use plain water and soft net or washcloth.
	  – wash from clean to dirty part of body (eyes to perineum).
	  – wash eyes from inner canthus to outer canthus.
	  – tub bathe baby 3 times/week after the cord falls off.
	  – do not apply lotions to infant's skin for 2 weeks.
	  – if desire to use powder, use one with a cornstarch base; apply with cotton balls.
	  – comb hair daily with a fine-toothed baby comb.
	7. Instruct on cord care
	  – clean around the cord with alcohol (on cotton balls) 3 times/daily or after each diaper change.
	  – small amounts of yellowish or serous bloody drainage is normal.

Mia Perrin   Admitting Diagnosis: Full-Term Pregnancy *(continued)*

Nursing Diagnosis	Expected Outcomes	Ongoing Assessment and Interventions	Outcome
		note drainage of any other color, foul-smelling drainage, or redness in cord area; call MD.	2. Correct return demonstrations of postpartum/newborn care
		8. Instruct on infant (female) perineal care	
		– small to moderate whitish or blood-tinged discharge is normal.	
		– when cleansing perineum, clean gently between labia, washing towards the rectum only.	
Potential alteration in parenting related to expressed fear and anxiety about inexperience with infants	*Target Date*: 2 days	1. Evaluate parent/child interactions.	1. Relaxed affect (parental) during parent/child interactions
	1. Parents will verbalize decreased fear and anxiety related to inexperience with infants.	2. Assess parents' learning needs.	
		3. Encourage parents to verbalize fears and anxiety, and to ask questions about childcare and development.	2. Appropriate parent/child interactions in specific situations
		4. Offer written information (e.g., pamphlets) about childcare and development.	3. Increased comfort with responsibility for an infant (confirmed by patient)
		5. Allow parents to spend time with their infant; provide support and reassurance about parent/child interaction.	

182   Nursing Diagnosis Care Plans

Knowledge deficit regarding infant stimulation needs/techniques	*Target Date:* 3 days
	1. Parents will verbalize and demonstrate knowledge of infant stimulation.
		1. Assess learner readiness.
		2. Provide information in small increments.
		3. Provide necessary reinforcements.
		4. Instruct on infant stimulation
		  – infant prefers upright position (place baby in infant seat).
		  – put mobiles in crib close to infant's face.
		  – use patterned sheets, bumper pads, and blankets.
		  – change the infant's environment during wakeful periods; move from room to room, take for a ride or walk.
		  – talk to, cuddle, and walk with the infant.
			4. Initiation of appropriate questions
			5. Active participation in infant care
			1. Confidence in knowledge of infant stimulation (confirmed by parents)
			2. Demonstration of appropriate interaction and infant stimulation

John Smith Admitting Diagnosis: Guillain-Barré Syndrome

Social History

Mr. Smith is a 71-year-old widowed male, a retired teacher, who lives in his own house with his son (the only living relative). Prior to this admission, he enjoyed a healthy, independent life-style with active involvement in church and social affairs.

History Present Illness

Approximately 1 month ago, Mr. Smith had an upper respiratory infection. The symptoms cleared spontaneously. Three days after resolution, Mr. Smith complained of bilateral numbness and tingling in his feet and ankles and associated difficulty walking. The numbness rapidly ascended over the following 36 hours, and Mr. Smith sought medical attention. On his admission to ICU, he could move nothing from his neck down, had difficulty talking and breathing; sensation existed only from his neck up. During the past 3 days, the numbness has been descending. He is now being transferred out of ICU, where he has been for the past 2 weeks.

Past Medical History

Essentially negative

Allergies

Penicillin

Physical Examination

Presentation

- Height 5 ft 6 in, weight 150 lb
- Alert and oriented to person, place, and time

- Speech slow and intermittently labored; no hoarseness
- Facial affect appropriate and tense; he states, "I'm mighty worried—I can't move or do anything for myself. What's going to happen to me?"

Skin
- No cyanosis; warm and dry; intact throughout
- Turgor elastic with rapid return

Eyes, Ears, Nose, Throat
- Pupils are equal, reactive to light and accommodation; extraocular movements are intact
- Conjuctiva clear; sclera white
- No discharge
- Oral mucosa moist, pink, and intact without lesions; full set of dentures in place
- Gag and cough reflexes present; chewing and swallowing actions normal
- Cervical nodes are nonpalpable

Cardiac
- Blood pressure 124/78, apical pulse 80/minute; regular rate and rhythm, without murmur
- Nailbed capillary refill less than 2 seconds
- Extremities are warm to touch

Respiratory
- Respirations are spontaneous and shallow at rate of 28/minute
- Even resonance bilaterally on percussion
- Auscultation reveals a few scattered rhonchi that clear with coughing

Admitting Diagnosis: Guillain-Barré Syndrome *(continued)*

- On demand, Mr. Smith is able to cough to produce small amounts of clear sputum

Gastrointestinal

- Abdomen soft, flat, nontender
- No palpable masses or nodes
- Last bowel movement 3 days ago; stool was hard, brown, and formed

Genitourinary

- Reports unawareness of urge to void, and is irregularly incontinent of varying amounts; needs to be straight catheterized 2–3 time/24 hours
- Urine is clear amber without foul odor

Neuromuscular

- Sensation level is at the costal margin
- No muscle atrophy in upper or lower extremities
- Active range of motion of the head, neck, and shoulders, as well as complete passive range of motion in all joints without tenderness or resistance
- Weak, gross motor movement of arms is present (bilaterally)—no fine motor movement in upper or lower extremities
- Aware of the position of upper extremities but is unaware of lower extremity position (bilaterally)
- Complains of tingling and numbness in upper extremities (no tingling below the costal margin); also complains of painful shoulders, unrelated to position or movement

Ineffective breathing pattern related to neuromuscular impairment	*Target Date:* 5 days	1. Assess and auscultate breath sounds every 4 hours and prn.	1. Clear breath sounds throughout all lung fields

	1. Patient's lungs will be clear to auscultation.	2. Monitor tissue perfusion
		  – nailbeds
		  – mucous membranes
		  – warmth of extremities
		  – edema.
			2. Even, unlabored respirations (16–20/ minute at rest)

	2. Respiration will be even and unlabored.	3. Monitor lab values and report significant changes
		  – ABGs
		  – chem. profile.
			3. No shortness of breath (confirmed by patient)

		4. Promote deep breathing, use of incentive spirometer every 2 hours while awake; have pt. cough to clear rhonchi after each series of deep breaths.	

		5. Instruct pt. and observe a return demonstration of adaptive breathing methods
		  – pursed-lip breathing
		  – slow, deep breaths
		  – use of accessory muscles.	

		6. Turn and reposition every 2 hours and prn.	
		7. Institute emergency measures if respiratory distress develops.	

JOHN SMITH   Admitting Diagnosis: GUILLAIN-BARRÉ SYNDROME *(continued)*

Nursing Diagnosis	Expected Outcomes	Ongoing Assessment and Interventions	Outcome
Potential alteration in skin integrity related to immobility, incontinence, and diaphoresis	*Target Date:* 10 days 1. Patient's skin will remain dry and intact.	1. Assess pressure points and skin integrity with every repositioning and with general assessment every shift. 2. Keep pt. on alternating pressure mattress when in bed. 3. Clean and dry skin promptly after diaphoresis and incontinence; provide change of linen prn. 4. Turn and reposition every 1–2 hours prn. 5. Massage pressure areas and bony prominences with lotion after every turning.	1. Skin intact; no redness 2. No discomfort related to skin breakdown (confirmed by patient)
Alteration in comfort: pain related to aching shoulders and generalized numbness and tingling	*Target Date:* 10 days 1. Patient's discomfort will decrease.	1. Assess – source of pain – intensity and location – alleviating and aggravating factors. 2. Change position every 1–2 hours and prn; use pillows to support back, head, and extremities.	1. Relaxed affect 2. Decreased discomfort (confirmed by patient) 3. Comfortable rest at night

Potential for injury related to neuromuscular impairment and possible paralysis	*Target Date*: 10 days
	1. Patient will remain free from injury.
	
	2. Patient's neuromuscular impairment will decrease or remain within baseline assessment.
		3. Encourage verbalization of pain and discomfort.
		4. Medicate for pain as needed; monitor for effectiveness.
		5. Utilize massage with physical therapy as scheduled and prn.
		1. Perform neurologic assessment every shift and prn
		  – level of consciousness and orientation
		  – pupils
		    • response to light
		    • extraocular movement
		    • peripheral vision
		  – sensory level
		    • light touch
		    • deep touch
		    • pain response
		    • position of extremities.
		2. Assess active range of motion every shift.
		3. Maintain correct body alignment every time pt. is turned and prn.
		4. Use correct lifting technique when moving pt.; do not pull on shoulders or legs; use two people.
			1. Range of motion (active and passive) remains within or improves from baseline assessment
			2. Tolerance for increased periods of active/passive range of motion
			3. Free from injury

JOHN SMITH   **Admitting Diagnosis: GUILLAIN-BARRÉ SYNDROME** *(continued)*

Nursing Diagnosis	Expected Outcomes	Ongoing Assessment and Interventions	Outcome

Potential fluid volume deficit related to high insensible fluid loss secondary to nerve impairment	*Target Date:* 10 days
	1. Patient will maintain fluid balance.
		5. Pad furniture and bony prominences.
		6. Keep call system and personal articles within easy reach.
		1. Assess every shift and prn
		  – mucous membranes
		  – skin turgor
		  – skin color
		  – skin temperature
		  – insensible fluid loss
		  – lung sounds (every 4 hours).
		2. Monitor level of consciousness.
		3. Accurately monitor and record I&O.
		4. Monitor and record vital signs every 4 hours and prn; do orthostatic vital signs bid.
		5. Obtain weight (in gown) at same time every morning.
			1. Warm, dry, elastic skin with intact, moist mucous membranes
			2. No excessive thirst; adequate urine output
			3. Balanced I&O
			4. Lab values within normal limits

Alteration in patterns of urinary elimination related to neuromuscular deficits	*Target Date:* 5 days
	1. Patient will establish an effective pattern of urinary elimination.
		6. Monitor lab values and report significant changes to MD.
		  – urinalysis, urine osmolarity, electrolytes, specific gravity
		  – chem profile, electrolytes
		  – BUN, creatinine.
		7. Encourage oral fluids to 2,000–2,500 cc/24 hours; pt. likes orange juice, soda pop, and popsicles.
		1. Perform abdominal assessment every shift.
		2. Palpate bladder gently every 2 hours.
		3. Monitor every 4 hours and prn
		  – I&O
		  – characteristics of urine
		  – perineal skin integrity
		  – restlessness.
		4. Place external catheter and connect to drainage bag for accurate I&O.
		5. Straight catheterize pt. every 4-6 hours prn bladder distention.
			1. Comfort and satisfaction with urinary elimination pattern (confirmed by patient)
			2. No bladder distention
			3. Balanced I&O
			4. Lab values within normal limits

JOHN SMITH Admitting Diagnosis: GUILLAIN-BARRÉ SYNDROME (continued)

Nursing Diagnosis	Expected Outcomes	Ongoing Assessment and Interventions	Outcome
		6. When in sitting position, as for therapy, encourage pt. to void. 7. Maintain consistent perineal care; keep clean and dry. 8. As pt.'s strength increases, begin bladder training per protocol.	
Self-care deficit (total) related to neuromuscular impairment	*Target Date:* 5-10 days 1. Patient will be as independent as possible in ADL. 2. Patient will be well groomed.	1. Assess ability to chew and swallow every shift. 2. Position in chair or, if in bed, in high-Fowler's for feeding; maintain position for at least 30 minutes after meals. 3. Feed small amounts of food at a time; let pt. set the pace.	1. Satiety with regular (assisted) feedings (confirmed by patient) 2. Progressing acquisition of adaptive feeding skills

3. Patient will establish regular bowel and bladder evacuation.	4. Consult other members of the health care team to provide and begin instruction in the use of adaptive equipment so pt. can feed self when strength begins to return.	3. Daily baths satisfy hygiene needs and personal standards (confirmed by patient)
	5. Assess pt.'s ability to use gross motor movement or upper extremities to assist with bathing.	4. Satisfaction with hair washing schedule and procedure (confirmed by patient)
	6. Assist with a daily bed bath; keep pt. warm and comfortable during the prodecure.	5. Uses arms to move washcloth, wash chest
	7. Wash hair every other day, per pt.'s request.	
	8. Allow pt. to participate, whenever possible, in bath schedule and procedure.	6. Well-groomed appearance: hair in place, nails trimmed and clean, good oral hygiene
	9. Provide oral hygiene before and after meals, at hs, and prn.	
	10. Comb hair at least bid and per request.	7. Satisfaction with grooming and appearance (confirmed by patient)
	11. Keep nails trimmed and filed; inspect daily for rough edges.	
	12. Assist with hand washing before meals and prn.	
	13. Assist with self-grooming as strength returns; provide instruction and adaptive equipment as necessary.	
	14. See also plan under *Alteration in patterns of urinary elimination.*	

JOHN SMITH   **Admitting Diagnosis: GUILLAIN-BARRÉ SYNDROME** *(continued)*

Nursing Diagnosis	Expected Outcomes	Ongoing Assessment and Interventions	Outcome
		15. Promote bowel elimination by establishing a regular elimination pattern – offer bedpan/commode 45 minutes after breakfast, every other day (odd days, to comply with usual pattern of elimination). – provide privacy. – if bowels to not move at regular intervals, give bisacodyl rectal suppository prn, chart response.	8. Acquisition of adaptive skills and participation in grooming 9. Establishment of an effective voiding pattern 10. Regular bowel evacuation, no constipation 11. Satisfaction with toileting habits (confirmed by patient)
Anxiety related to immobility and inability to care for self secondary to neuromuscular impairment and the uncertainty of recovery potential	*Target Date:* 5 days 1. Patient will verbalize feelings. 2. Patient will accept explanations and participate in tasks to alleviate anxiety.	1. Identify the intensity of the anxiety, aggravating and alleviating factors. 2. Encourage pt. to verbalize feelings: listen when he talks about his anxieties and accept the validity of his feelings. 3. Offer reassurance and support, but do not foster false hope. 4. Keep environment quiet and comfortable, especially when pt. is fearful	

		5. Provide continuity of care. 6. Explain all tasks and procedures accurately at pt.'s level of understanding; provide accurate information on the disease process and on his progress; include son in as many explanations as possible. 7. Provide a reliable call system and answer calls promptly; anticipate needs when possible.	
		1. Open expression of feelings 2. Increased understanding of the disease process and progress toward recovery (confirmed by patient) 3. Relaxed affect 4. Increased comfort and awareness of what is happening (confirmed by patient)	
Powerlessness related to impaired physical control, lengthy hospitalization, and dependence on others	*Target Date:* 10 days 1. Patient will participate in decision making and completing tasks.	1. Assess pt.'s feelings of lack of control over self and environment. 2. Listen to verbal and nonverbal clues about feelings of powerlessness. 3. Encourage pt. to talk about his successes in life. 4. Encourage the son to include pt. in discussions of household and family matters and related decision making.	1. Active participation in decision making with family, staff, and friends 2. Completion of tasks resulting from independent decisions

John Smith **Admitting Diagnosis: Guillain-Barré Syndrome** *(continued)*

Nursing Diagnosis	Expected Outcomes	Ongoing Assessment and Interventions	Outcome
		5. Invite friends and fellow church members to visit and involve pt. (as his condition allows) in discussions and group decisions. 6. Reduce environmental stress. 7. Spend time with pt. every day exploring strengths and potential, encouraging participation in determining daily activity schedule. 8. Praise pt. progress in completing tasks and decisions.	

Bibliography

Armstrong, M., et al. (Eds.). (1979). *McGraw-Hill handbook of clinical nursing*. New York: McGraw-Hill.

Brunner, L., & Suddarth, D. (1982). *The Lippincott manual of nursing practice* (3rd ed.). Philadelphia: Lippincott.

Campbell, C. (1978). *Nursing diagnosis and intervention in nursing practice*. New York: Wiley.

Carpenito, L. (1984). *Handbook of nursing diagnosis*. Philadelphia: Lippincott.

Chatton, M. (Ed.). (1979). *Handbook of medical treatment*. (16th ed.). Greenbrae: Jones Medical Publications.

Coleman, J., & Hammer, C. (1974). *Contemporary psychology and effective behavior*. Glenview: Scott, Foresman.

Freitag, J., & Miller, L. (Eds.). (1980). *Manual of medical therapeutics*. Boston: Little, Brown.

Gettrust, K., Ryan, S., & Engelman, D. (Eds.). (1985). *Applied nursing diagnosis*. New York: Wiley.

Gordon, M. (1982). *Manual of nursing diagnosis*. New York: McGraw-Hill.

Hymovich, D., & Barnard, M. (Eds.). (1979). *Family health care—General perspectives* (Vol. 1). New York: McGraw-Hill.

Kim, M., McFarland, G., & McLane, A. (Eds.). (1984). *Pocket guide to nursing diagnoses*. St. Louis: Mosby.

Kübler-Ross, E. (1970). *On death and dying*. New York: Macmillan.

Little, D., & Carnevali, D. (1969). *Nursing care planning*. Philadelphia: Lippincott.

McEntyre, R. (1980). *Practical guide to the care of the surgical patient*. St. Louis: Mosby.

Rich, P. Make the most of your charting time. *Nursing 83, 13* (3), 34–39.

Smitherman, C. (1981). *Nursing actions for health promotion*. Philadelphia: F.A. Davis.

Wilson, H., & Kneisl, C. (1979). *Psychiatric nursing*. Menlo Park: Addison-Wesley.